# NLN PAX
# Test Prep

A Complete NLN PAX Study Guide
and Practice Test Questions

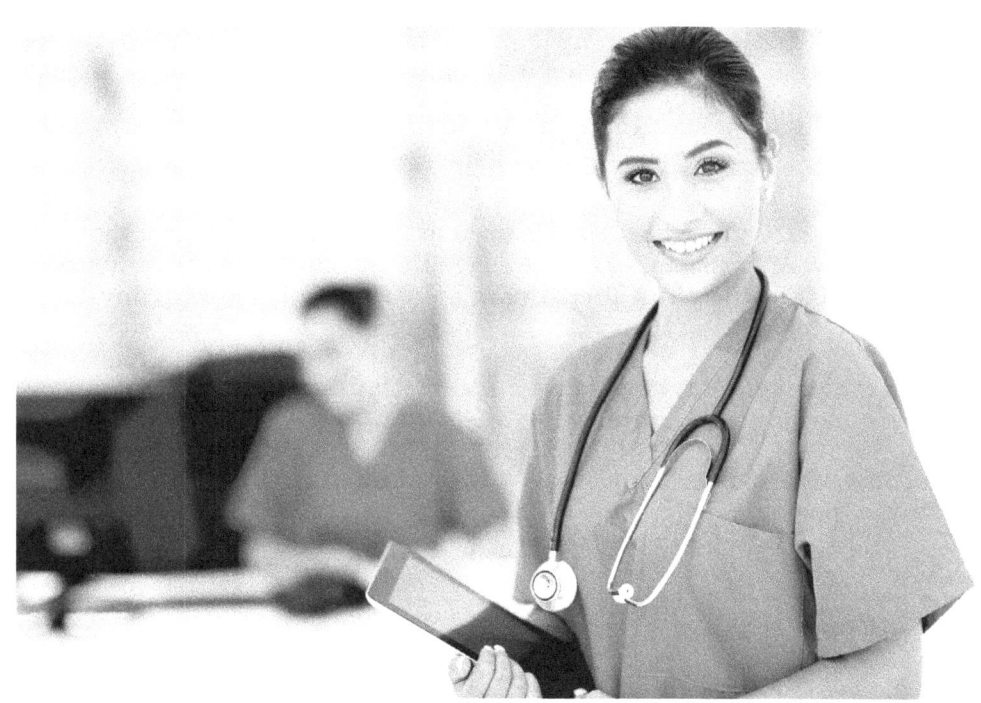

**COMPLETE**
Test Preparation Inc.
www.test-preparation.ca

Copyright © 2020 Complete Test Preparation Inc. ALL RIGHTS RESERVED.

No part of this book may be reproduced or transferred in any form or by any means, graphic, electronic, or mechanical, including photocopying, recording, web distribution, taping, or by any information storage retrieval system, without the written permission of the author.

Notice: Complete Test Preparation Inc. makes every reasonable effort to obtain from reliable sources accurate, complete, and timely information about the tests covered in this book. Nevertheless, changes can be made in the tests or the administration of the tests at any time and Complete Test Preparation Inc. makes no representation or warranty, either expressed or implied as to the accuracy, timeliness, or completeness of the information contained in this book. Complete Test Preparation Inc. makes no representations or warranties of any kind, express or implied, about the completeness, accuracy, reliability, suitability or availability with respect to the information contained in this document for any purpose. Any reliance you place on such information is therefore strictly at your own risk.

The author(s) shall not be liable for any loss incurred as a consequence of the use and application, directly or indirectly, of any information presented in this work. Sold with the understanding, the author is not engaged in rendering professional services or advice. If advice or expert assistance is required, the services of a competent professional should be sought.

The company, product and service names used in this publication are for identification purposes only. All trademarks and registered trademarks are the property of their respective owners. Complete Test Preparation Inc. is not affiliated with any educational institution.

**We strongly recommend that students check with exam providers for up-to-date information regarding test content.**

Please note that PAX RN is administered by the National League of Nursing which is not involved in the production of, and does not endorse, this product.

Version 9 June 2025

ISBN-13: 978-1-77245-523-6

# About Complete Test Preparation Inc.

**Why Us?**
The Complete Test Preparation Team has been publishing high quality study materials since 2005, with a catalogue of over 145 titles, in English, French and Chinese, as well as curriculum for all levels.

To keep up with the industry changes, we update everything all the time!

**And the best part?**
With every purchase, you're helping people all over the world improve themselves and their education. So thank you in advance for supporting this mission with us! Together, we are truly making a difference in the lives of those often forgotten by the system.

Charities that we support -
https://www.test-preparation.ca/charities-and-non-profits/

**You have definitely come to the right place.**
If you want to spend your valuable study time where it will help you the most - we've got you covered today and tomorrow.


Published by
Complete Test Preparation Inc.
Victoria BC Canada

Visit us on the web at https://www.test-preparation.ca
Printed in the USA


# Feedback

We welcome your feedback. Email us at feedback@test-preparation.ca with your comments and suggestions. We carefully review all suggestions and often incorporate reader suggestions into upcoming versions. As a Print on Demand Publisher, we update our products frequently.

# CONTENTS

**Getting Started**
    How this study guide is organized      6
    The PAX RN Study Plan      7
    Making a Study Schedule      9

**Verbal Ability**
    Self Assessment      14
    Answer Key      23
    Help with Reading Comprehension      26
    Main Idea, Topic and Supporting Details      28
    Drawing Inferences And Conclusions      32
    Meaning From Context      34
    Help with Building your Vocabulary      36

**Mathematics**
    Mathematics Self-Assessment      43
    Answer Key      50
    Basic Math Video Tutorials      55
    Fraction Tips, Tricks and Shortcuts      55
    Decimal Tips, Tricks and Short-cuts      58
    Converting Decimals to Fractions      58
    Percent Tips, Tricks and Shortcuts      59
    How to Answer Basic Math Multiple Choice      60
    How to Solve Word Problems      63
    Types of Word Problems      65
    Mean, Median and Mode      73
    Order Of Operation      74
    Scientific Notation      75
    Ratios      76
    Perimeter Area and Volume      79
    Area of Complex 2-D and 3-D Shapes      84
    Pythagorean Geometry      86
    Adding and Subtracting Polynomials      88
    Multiplying and Dividing Polynomials      88
    Simplifying Polynomials      89
    Factoring Polynomials      89
    Quadratic equations      90
    Momentum      91

**Science**
    Self-Assessment      101
    Answer Key      104
    Science Tutorials      108
    Scientific Method      108
    Cell Biology      110
    Chromosomes, genes, proteins, RNA and DNA      113

| | |
|---|---|
| Mitosis and Meiosis | 115 |
| Phenotypes and Genotypes | 116 |
| Heredity: Genes and Mutation | 119 |
| Heredity: Mendelian Inheritance | 120 |
| Classification | 122 |
| Ecology | 124 |
| Basic Concepts in Chemistry | 128 |
| Basic Physics | 139 |
| Energy: Work and Power | 142 |
| Defining Force and Newton's Three Laws | 144 |
| Force: Friction | 145 |
| Fundamental Forces: Electromagnetism | 146 |
| Fundamental Forces: Gravity | 148 |
| Fundamental Forces: Strong and Weak Nuclear Forces | 149 |
| Quantum Mechanics | 151 |
| States of Matter | 154 |
| Speed, Acceleration and Force Problems | 156 |

**Practice Test Questions Set 1**
Answer Key                                                                 200

**Practice Test Questions Set 2**
Answer Key                                                                 256

**Bonus Tests 3 and 4**

**Conclusion**

**Online Resources**

# Getting Started

CONGRATULATIONS! By deciding to take the Registered Nursing Program (PAX RN) Exam, you have taken the first step toward a great future! Of course, there is no point in taking this important examination unless you intend to do your best to earn the highest grade you possibly can. That means getting yourself organized and discovering the best approaches, methods and strategies to master the material. Yes, that will require real effort and dedication, but if you are willing to focus your energy and devote the study time necessary, before you know it you will be opening that letter of acceptance to the school of your dreams.

We know that taking on a new endeavour can be scary, and it is easy to feel unsure of where to begin. That's where we come in. This study guide is designed to help you improve your test-taking skills, show you a few tricks of the trade and increase both your competency and confidence.

## The Registered Nursing Program PAX Exam

The PAX RN Modules are: Mathematics, Verbal Ability (Reading Comprehension and Vocabulary), and Science which includes, Biology, Chemistry, Physics, Basic Scientific principals and Earth Science.

While we seek to make our guide as comprehensive as possible, note that like all entrance exams, the PAX RN Exam might be adjusted at some future point. New material might be added, or content that is no longer relevant or applicable might be removed. It is always a good idea to give the materials you receive when you register to take the PAX RN a careful review.

## How this study guide is organized

This study guide is divided into three sections. The first section, Self-Assessments, which will help you recognize your areas of strength and weaknesses. This will be a boon when it comes to managing your study time most efficiently; there is not much point of focusing on material you have already got firmly under control. Instead, taking the self-assessments will show you where that time could be much better spent. In this area you will begin with a few questions to evaluate quickly your understanding of material that is likely to appear on the PAX RN. If you do poorly in certain areas, simply work carefully through those sections in the tutorials and then try the self-assessment again.

The second section, Tutorials, offers information in each of the content areas, as well as strategies to help you master that material. The tutorials are not intended to be a complete course, but cover general principles. If you find that you do not understand the tutorials, it is recommended that you seek out additional instruction. Most Universities recommend student take introductory courses in Math, English and Science before taking the PAX RN.

Third, we offer two sets of practice test questions, similar to those on the PAX RN Exam. Again, we cover all modules, so make sure to check with your school!

Besides all these materials, the last three chapters give you important information on how to answer multiple choice questions, how to prepare for a test, and how to take a test.

## The PAX Study Plan

Now that you have made the decision to take the PAX RN, it is time to get started. Before you do another thing, you will need to figure out a plan of attack. The very best study tip is to start early! The longer the time period you devote to regular study practice, the likelier you will be to retain the material and access it quickly. If you thought that 1 x 20 is the same as 2 x 10, guess what? It really is not, when it comes to study time. Reviewing material for just an hour per day over the course of 20 days is far better than studying for two hours a day for only 10 days. The more often you revisit a particular piece of information, the better you will know it. Not only will your grasp and understanding be better, but your ability to reach into your brain and quickly and efficiently pull out the tidbit you need, will be greatly enhanced as well.

The great Chinese scholar and philosopher Confucius believed that true knowledge could be defined as knowing what you know and what you do not know. The first step in preparing for the PAX RN Exam is to assess your strengths and weaknesses. You may already have an idea of what you know and what you do not know, but evaluating yourself using our Self- Assessment modules for each of the three areas, Math, Science and Verbal Ability, will clarify the details.

## Making a Study Schedule

To make your study time the most productive, you will need to develop a study plan. The purpose of the plan is to organize all the bits of pieces of information in such a way that you will not feel overwhelmed. Rome was not built in a day, and learning everything you will need to know to pass the PAX RN Exam is going to take time, too. Arranging the material you need to learn into manageable chunks is the best way to go. Each study session should make you feel as though you have accomplished your goal, or at least are closer, and your goal is simply to learn what you planned to learn during that particular session. Try to organize the content in such a way that each study session builds on previous ones. That way, you will retain the information, be better able to access it, and review the previous bits and pieces at the same time.

## Self-assessment

**The Best Study Tip!** The very best study tip is to start early! The longer you study regularly, the more you will retain and 'learn' the material. Studying for 1 hour per day for 20 days is far better than studying for 2 hours for 10 days.

**What don't you know?**

The first step is to assess your strengths and weaknesses. You may already have an idea of where your weaknesses are, or you can take our Self-assessment modules for each of the areas, Math, Science and Verbal Ability.

| Exam Component | Rate 1 to 5 |
| --- | --- |
| **Verbal Ability** | |
| | |
| Paragraph & Passage Comprehension | |
| Vocabulary | |
| **Math** | |
| Fractions, Decimals, Percent | |
| Word Problems | |
| Percent | |
| Median and Mode | |
| Scientific Notation | |
| Quadratics and Polynomials | |
| Speed and Momentum | |
| Basic Algebra | |
| **Science** | |
| Biology | |
| Physics | |
| Earth Science | |
| Chemistry | |

## Making a Study Schedule

The key to making a study plan is to divide the material you need to learn into manageable size and learn it, while at the same time reviewing the material that you already know.

Using the table above, any scores of 3 or below, you need to spend time learning, reviewing and practicing this subject area. A score of 4 means you need to review the material, but you don't have to re-learn it. A score of 5 and you are OK with just an occasional review before the exam.

A score of 0 or 1 means you really need to work on this area and should allocate the most time and the highest priority. Some students prefer a 5-day plan and others a 10-day plan. It also depends on how much time until the exam.

Here is an example of a 5-day plan based on an example from the table above:

Fractions: 1  Study 1 hour everyday – review on last day
Biology: 3  Study 1 hour for 2 days then ½ hour a day, then review
Vocabulary: 4  Review every second day
Word Problems: 2 Study 1 hour on the first day – then ½ hour everyday
Reading Comprehension: 5  Review for ½ hour every other day
Algebra: 5  Review for ½ hour every other day
Chemistry: 5 very confident – review a few times.

Based on this, here is a sample study plan:

| Day | Subject | Time |
|---|---|---|
| | | |
| **Monday** | | |
| Study | Fractions | 1 hour |
| Study | Word Problems | 1 hour |
| | **½ hour break** | |
| Study | Biology | 1 hour |
| Review | Chemistry | ½ hour |
| | | |
| **Tuesday** | | |
| Study | Fractions | 1 hour |
| Study | Word Problems | ½ hour |
| | **½ hour break** | |
| Study | Decimals | ½ hour |
| Review | Vocabulary | ½ hour |
| Review | Grammar | ½ hour |
| | | |

| Wednesday | | |
|---|---|---|
| Study | Fractions | 1 hour |
| Study | Word Problems | ½ hour |
| | **½ hour break** | |
| Study | Biology | ½ hour |
| Review | Chemistry | ½ hour |
| | | |
| **Thursday** | | |
| Study | Fractions | ½ hour |
| Study | Word Problems | ½ hour |
| Review | Biology | ½ hour |
| | **½ hour break** | |
| Review | Grammar | ½ hour |
| Review | Vocabulary | ½ hour |
| | | |
| **Friday** | | |
| Review | Fractions | ½ hour |
| Review | Word Problems | ½ hour |
| Review | Biology | ½ hour |
| | **½ hour break** | |
| Review | Vocabulary | ½ hour |
| Review | Grammar | ½ hour |

# Verbal Ability

This section contains a self-assessment and reading tutorial. The Tutorials are designed to familiarize general principles and the self-assessment contains general questions similar to the reading questions likely to be on the PAX RN exam, but are not intended to be identical to the exam questions. The tutorials are not designed to be a complete reading course, and it is assumed that students have some familiarity with Verbal Ability questions. If you do not understand parts of the tutorial, or find the tutorial difficult, it is recommended that you seek out additional instruction.

## Tour of the PAX RN Reading Content

The PAX RN reading section has 47 questions that must be answered in 60 minutes. Below is a more detailed list of the types of reading questions that generally appear on the PAX RN.

- Drawing logical conclusions
- Identifying main ideas
- Meaning in context
- Distinguish fact from opinions
- Making inferences
- Identifying tone and purpose
- Summarizing

The questions below are not the same as you will find on the PAX RN - that would be too easy! And nobody knows what the questions will be and they change all the time. Mostly the changes consist of substituting new questions for old, but the changes can be new question formats or styles, changes to the number of questions in each section, changes to the time limits for each section and combining sections. Below are general reading questions that cover the same areas as the PAX RN. So, while the format and exact wording of the questions may differ slightly, and change from year to year, if you can answer the questions below, you will have no problem with the verbal ability section of the PAX RN.

## Reading Self-Assessment

The purpose of the self-assessment is:

- Identify your strengths and weaknesses.
- Develop your personalized study plan (above)
- Get accustomed to the PAX RN format
- Extra practice – the self-assessments are almost a full 3rd practice test!
- Provide a baseline score for preparing your study schedule.

Since this is a Self-assessment, and depending on how confident you are with Verbal Ability, timing is optional. The PAX RN has 80 reading questions including vocabulary. The self-assessment has 40 questions, so allow about 45 minutes to complete this assessment.

Once complete, use the table below to assess your understanding of the content, and prepare your study schedule described in chapter 1.

For additional help with answering multiple choice reading comprehension questions, see www.multiple-choice.ca

| 80% - 100% | Excellent – you have mastered the content |
|---|---|
| 60 – 79% | Good. You have a working knowledge. Even though you can just pass this section, you may want to review the tutorials and do some extra practice to see if you can improve your mark. |
| 40% - 59% | Below Average. You do not understand the Verbal Ability problems.<br><br>Review the tutorials, and retake this quiz again in a few days, before proceeding to the rest of the study guide. |
| Less than 40% | Poor. You have a very limited understanding of the Verbal Ability problems.<br><br>Please review the tutorials, and retake this quiz again in a few days, before proceeding to the rest of the study guide. |

# Verbal Ability Self-Assessment Answer Sheet

1. A B C D    11. A B C D    21. A B C D    31. A B C D
2. A B C D    12. A B C D    22. A B C D    32. A B C D
3. A B C D    13. A B C D    23. A B C D    33. A B C D
4. A B C D    14. A B C D    24. A B C D    34. A B C D
5. A B C D    15. A B C D    25. A B C D    35. A B C D
6. A B C D    16. A B C D    26. A B C D    36. A B C D
7. A B C D    17. A B C D    27. A B C D    37. A B C D
8. A B C D    18. A B C D    28. A B C D    38. A B C D
9. A B C D    19. A B C D    29. A B C D    39. A B C D
10. A B C D   20. A B C D    30. A B C D    40. A B C D

**Questions 1 – 4 refer to the following passage.**

**Passage 1 - Who Was Anne Frank?**

You may have heard mention of the word Holocaust in your History or English classes. The Holocaust took place from 1939-1945. It was an attempt by the Nazi party to purify the human race, by eliminating Jews, Gypsies, Catholics, homosexuals and others they deemed inferior to their "perfect" Aryan race. The Nazis used Concentration Camps, which were sometimes used as Death Camps, to exterminate the people they held in the camps. The saddest fact about the Holocaust was the over one million children under the age of sixteen died in a Nazi concentration camp. Just a few weeks before World War II was over, Anne Frank was one of those children to die.

Before the Nazi party began its persecution of the Jews, Anne Frank had a happy life. She was born in June of 1929. In June of 1942, for her 13th birthday, she was given a simple present which would go onto impact the lives of millions of people around the world. That gift was a small red diary that she called Kitty. This diary was to become Anne's most treasured possession when she and her family hid from the Nazis in a secret annex above her father's office building in Amsterdam.

For 25 months, Anne, her sister Margot, her parents, another family, and an elderly Jewish dentist hid from the Nazis in this tiny annex. They were never permitted to go outside, and their food and supplies were brought to them by Miep Gies and her husband, who did not believe in the Nazi persecution of the Jews. It was a very difficult life for young Anne and she used Kitty as an outlet to describe her life in hiding. After 2 years, Anne and her family were betrayed and arrested by the Nazis. To this day, nobody is exactly sure who betrayed the Frank family and the other annex residents. Anne, her mother, and her sister were separated from Otto Frank, Anne's father. Then, Anne and Margot were separated from their mother. In March of 1945, Margot Frank died of starvation in a Concentration Camp. A few days later, at the age of 15, Anne Frank died of typhus. Of all the people who hid in the Annex, only Otto Frank survived the Holocaust.

Otto Frank returned to the Annex after World War II. It was there that he found Kitty, filled with Anne's thoughts and feelings about being a persecuted Jewish girl. Otto Frank had Anne's diary published in 1947 and it has remained continuously in print ever since. Today, the diary has been published in over 55 languages and more than 24 million copies have been sold around the world. The Diary of Anne Frank tells the story of a brave young woman who tried to see the good in all people.

**1. From the context clues in the passage, what does annex mean?**

    a. Attic

    b. Bedroom

    c. Basement

    d. Kitchen

**2. Why do you think Anne's diary has been published in 55 languages?**

    a. So everyone could understand it.

    b. So people around the world could learn more about the horrors of the Holocaust.

    c. Because Anne was Jewish but hid in Amsterdam and died in Germany.

    d. Because Otto Frank spoke many languages.

**3. From the description of Anne and Margot's deaths in the passage, what can we assume typhus is?**

    a. The same as starving to death.

    b. An infection the Germans gave to Anne.

    c. A disease Anne caught in the concentration camp.

    d. Poison gas used by the Germans to kill Anne.

**4. In the third paragraph, what does outlet mean?**

    a. A place to plug things into the wall

    b. A store where Miep bought cheap supplies for the Frank family

    c. A hiding space similar to an Annex

    d. A place where Anne could express her private thoughts.

**Questions 5 – 8 refer to the following passage.**

**Passage 2 - Was Dr. Seuss A Real Doctor?**

A favorite author for over 100 years, Theodor Seuss Geisel was born on March 2, 1902. Today, we celebrate the birthday of the famous "Dr. Seuss" by hosting Read Across America events throughout the March. School children around the country celebrate the "Doctor's" birthday by making hats, giving presentations and holding read aloud circles featuring some of Dr. Seuss' most famous books.

But who was Dr. Seuss? Did he go to medical school? Where was his office? You may be surprised to know that Theodor Seuss Geisel was not a medical doctor at all. He took on the nickname Dr. Seuss when he became a noted children's book author. He earned the nickname because people said his books were "as good as medicine." All these years later, his nickname has lasted and he is known as Dr. Seuss all across the world.

Think back to when you were a young child. Did you ever want to try "green eggs and ham?" Did you try to "Hop on Pop?" Do you remember learning about the environment from a creature called The Lorax? Of course, you must recall one of Seuss' most famous characters; that green Grinch who stole Christmas. These stories were all written by Dr. Seuss and featured his signature rhyming words and letters. They also featured made up words to enhance his rhyme scheme and even though many of his characters were made up, they sure seem real to us today.

And what of his "signature" book, The Cat in the Hat? You must remember that cat and Thing One and Thing Two from your childhood. Did you know that in the early 1950's there was a growing concern in America that children were not becoming avid readers? This was, book publishers thought, because children found books dull and uninteresting. An intelligent publisher sent Dr. Seuss a book of words that he thought all children should learn as young readers. Dr. Seuss wrote his famous story The Cat in the Hat, using those words. We can see, over the decades, just how much influence his writing has had on very young children. That is why we celebrate this doctor's birthday each March.

**5. What does the word "avid" mean in the last paragraph?**

   a. Good

   b. Interested

   c. Slow

   d. Fast

**6. What can we infer from the statement " His books were like medicine?"**

   a. His books made people feel better

   b. His books were in doctor's office waiting rooms

   c. His books took away fevers

   d. His books left a funny taste in readers' mouths.

**7. Why is the publisher in the last paragraph called "intelligent?"**

   a. The publisher knew how to read.

   b. The publisher knew that kids did not like to read.

   c. The publisher knew Dr. Seuss would be able to create a book that sold well.

   d. The publisher knew that Dr. Seuss would be able to write a book that would get young children interested in reading.

**8. The theme of this passage is**

   a. Dr. Seuss was not a doctor.

   b. Dr. Seuss influenced the lives of generations of young children.

   c. Dr. Seuss wrote rhyming books.

   d. Dr. Seuss' birthday is a good day to read a book.

**Questions 9 - 12 refer to the following passage.**

**Keeping Tropical Fish**

Keeping tropical fish at home or in your office used to be very popular. Today, interest has declined, but it remains as rewarding and relaxing a hobby as ever. Ask any tropical fish hobbyist, and you will hear how soothing and relaxing watching colorful fish live their lives in the aquarium. If you are considering keeping tropical fish as pets, here is a list of basic equipment you will need.

A filter is essential for keeping your aquarium clean and your fish alive and healthy. There are different types and sizes of filters and the right size for you depends on the size of the aquarium and the level of stocking. Generally, you need a filter with a 3 to 5 times turn over rate per hour. This means that the water in the tank should go through the filter about 3 to 5 times per hour.

Most tropical fish do well in water temperatures ranging between $24^0$ C and $26^0$ C, though each has its own ideal water temperature. A heater with a thermostat is necessary to regulate the water temperature. Some heaters are submersible and others are not, so check carefully before you buy.

Lights are also necessary, and come in a large variety of types, strengths and sizes. A light source is necessary for plants in the tank to photosynthesize and give the tank a more attractive appearance. Even if you plan to use plastic plants, the fish still require light, although here you can use a lower strength light source.

A hood is necessary to keep dust, dirt and unwanted materials out of the tank. Sometimes the hood can also help prevent evaporation. Another requirement is aquarium gravel. This will improve the aesthetics of the aquarium and is necessary if you plan to have real plants.

**9. What is the general tone of this article?**

   a. Formal
   b. Informal
   c. Technical
   d. Opinion

**10. Which of the following cannot be inferred?**

   a. Gravel is good for aquarium plants.
   b. Fewer people have aquariums in their office than at home.
   c. The larger the tank, the larger the filter required.
   d. None of the above.

**11. What evidence does the author provide to support their claim that aquarium lights are necessary?**

a. Plants require light.
b. Fish and plants require light.
c. The author does not provide evidence for this statement.
d. Aquarium lights make the aquarium more attractive.

**12. Which of the following is an opinion?**

a. Filter with a 3 to 5 times turn over rate per hour are required.
b. Aquarium gravel improves the aesthetics of the aquarium.
c. An aquarium hood keeps dust, dirt and unwanted materials out of the tank.
d. Each type of tropical fish has its own ideal water temperature.

**Questions 13 - 15 refer to the following passage.**

**The Civil War**

The Civil War began on April 12, 1861. The first shots of the Civil War were fired in Fort Sumter, South Carolina. Even though more American lives were lost in the Civil War than in any other war, not one person died on that first day. The war began because eleven Southern states seceded from the Union and tried to start their own government, The Confederate States of America.

Why did the states secede? The issue of slavery was a primary cause of the Civil War. The eleven southern states relied heavily on their slaves to foster their farming and plantation lifestyles. The northern states, many of whom had already abolished slavery, did not think that the southern states should have slaves. The north wanted to free all the slaves and President Lincoln's goal was to both end slavery and preserve the Union. He had Congress declare war on the Confederacy on April 14, 1862. For four long, blood soaked years, the North and South fought.

From 1861 to mid 1863, it seemed as if the South would win this war. However, on July 1, 1863, an epic three day battle was waged on a field in Gettysburg, Pennsylvania. Gettysburg is remembered for being the bloodiest battle in American history. At the end of the three days, the North turned the tide of the war in their favor. The North then went on to dominate the South for the remainder of the war. Another famous event is General Sherman's "March to The Sea," where he famously led the Union Army through Georgia and the Carolinas, burning and destroying everything in their path.
In 1865, the Union army invaded and captured the Confederate capital of Richmond Virginia. Robert E. Lee, leader of the Confederacy surrendered to General Ulysses S. Grant, leader of the Union forces, on April 9, 1865. The Civil War was over and the Union was preserved.

**13. What does secede mean?**

    a. To break away from

    b. To accomplish

    c. To join

    d. To lose

**14. Which of the following statements summarizes a FACT from the passage?**

    a. Congress declared war and then the Battle of Fort Sumter began.

    b. Congress declared war after shots were fired at Fort Sumter.

    c. President Lincoln was pro slavery

    d. President Lincoln was at Fort Sumter with Congress

**15. Which event finally led the Confederacy to surrender?**

    a. The battle of Gettysburg

    b. The battle of Bull Run

    c. The invasion of the confederate capital of Richmond

    d. Sherman's March to the Sea

## Part II – Vocabulary

**16. Choose the noun that means, self-evident or clear obvious truth.**

   a. Truism
   b. Catharsis
   c. Libertine
   d. Tractable

**17. Choose the best definition for: virago**

   a. A loud domineering woman
   b. A quiet woman
   c. A load domineering Man
   d. A quiet man

**18. When Joe broke his _____ in a skiing accident, his entire leg was in a cast.**

   a. Ankle
   b. Humerus
   c. Wrist
   d. Femur

**19. Select another word for the underlined word in the sentence below.**

**At first I thought she was very rude and boorish, but when I talked to her again she was very genteel.**

   a. Chivalrous
   b. Hilarious
   c. Civilized
   d. Governance

**20. Choose an adjective that means corrupted, impure.**

   a. Adulterate
   b. Harbor
   c. Infuriate
   d. Inculcate

**21. Select another word for the underlined word in the sentence below.**

**Her business success showed that she was very shrewd.**

   a. Slow
   b. Astute
   c. Ignorant
   d. Heinous

**22. Choose an adjective that means, beyond what is obvious or evident.**

   a. Ulterior
   b. Sybarite
   c. Torsion
   d. Trenchant

**23. Choose a noun that means, homeless child or stray.**

   a. Elegy
   b. Waif
   c. Martyr
   d. Palaver

**24. Select another word for the underlined word in the sentence below.**

**His inheritance was very large - a princely sum!**

   a. Minor
   b. Tolerable
   c. Large
   d. Pittance

**25. What is the best definition of deprecate?**

   a. Approve
   b. Indifference
   c. Disapprove
   d. None of the above

**26. Choose the best definition for succor.**

   a. To suck on
   b. To hate
   c. To like
   d. Give help of assistance

**27. Select the synonym of conspicuous.**

   a. Important
   b. Prominent
   c. Beautiful
   d. Convincing

**28. Select the noun that means eagerness and enthusiasm.**

   a. Alacrity
   b. Happiness
   c. Donator
   d. Marital

**29. Fill in the blank.**

**After Lisa's aunt had her tenth child, Lisa found that she had more than twenty _____.**

   a. Uncles
   b. Friends
   c. Stepsisters
   d. Cousins

**30. Select the word that means benevolence.**

   a. Happiness
   b. Courage
   c. Kindness
   d. Loyalty

**31. Select the verb that means, to make less severe.**

   a. Suspense
   b. Alleviate
   c. Ingrate
   d. Action

**32. What is the name of one who gives a gift or who gives money to a charity organization?**

   a. Captain
   b. Benefactor
   c. Source
   d. Teacher

33. What is another word for subordinate, or person of lesser rank or authority?

    a. Palliate

    b. Plebeian

    c. Underling

    d. Expiate

34. Choose the best definition of specious.

    a. Logical

    b. Illogical

    c. Emotional

    d. 2 species

35. Choose the best definition of proscribe.

    a. Welcome

    b. Write a prescription

    c. Banish

    d. Give a diagnosis

36. Fill in the blank.

When Craig's dog was struck by a car, he rushed his pet to the _____.

    a. Emergency room

    b. Doctor

    c. Veterinarian

    d. Podiatrist

37. Select another word for the underlined word in the sentence below.
She never made a mistake - her performance was always <u>impeccable</u>.

    a. Charming

    b. Flattering

    c. Perfect

    d. Impervious

38. Select the synonym of boisterous.

    a. Loud

    b. Soft

    c. Gentle

    d. Warm

39. Select the adjective that means hidden, secret, disguised.

    a. Accustomed

    b. Covert

    c. Hide

    d. Carriage

40. Select the verb that means straightforward, open and sincere.

    a. Lawful

    b. Candid

    c. True

    d. Lawful

## Answer Key

**1. A**

We know that an annex is like an attic because the text states the annex was above Otto Frank's building.

Choice B is incorrect because an office building doesn't have bedrooms. Choice C is incorrect because a basement would be below the office building. Choice D is incorrect because there would not be a kitchen in an office building.

**2. B**

The diary has been published in 55 languages so people all over the world can learn about Anne. That is why the passage says it has been continuously in print.

Choice A is incorrect because it is too vague. Choice C is incorrect because it was published after Anne died and she did not write in all three languages. Choice D is incorrect because the passage does not give us any information about what languages Otto Frank spoke.

**3. C**

Use the process of elimination to figure this out.

Choice A cannot be the correct answer because, otherwise the passage would have simply said that Anne and Margot both died of starvation. Choices B and D cannot be correct because, if the Germans had done something specifically to murder Anne, the passage would have stated that directly. By the process of elimination, choice C has to be the correct answer.

**4. D**

We can figure this out using context clues. The paragraph is talking about Anne's diary and so, outlet in this instance is a place where Anne can pour her feelings.

Choice A is incorrect answer. That is the literal meaning of the word outlet and the passage is using the figurative meaning. Choice B is incorrect because that is the secondary literal meaning of the word outlet, as in an outlet mall. Again, we are looking for figurative meaning. Choice C is incorrect because there are no clues in the text to support that answer.

**5. B**

When someone is avid about something that means they are highly interested in the subject. The context clues are dull and boring, because they define the opposite of avid.

**6. A**

The author is using a simile to compare the books to medicine. Medicine is what you take when you want to feel better. They are suggesting that if you want to feel good, they should read Dr. Seuss' books.

Choice B is incorrect because there is no mention of a doctor's office. Choice C is incorrect because it is using the literal meaning of medicine and the author is using medicine in a figurative way. Choice D is incorrect because it makes no sense. We know not to eat books.

**7. D**

The publisher is described as intelligent because he knew to get in touch with a famous author to develop a book that children would be interested in reading.

Choice A is incorrect because we can assume that all book publishers must know how to read. Choice B is incorrect because it says in the article that more than one publisher was concerned whether children liked to read. Choice D is incorrect because there is no mention in the article about how well The Cat in the Hat sold when it was first published.

**8. B**

The passage describes in detail how Dr. Seuss had a great effect on the lives of children through his writing. It names several of his books, tells how he helped children become avid readers and explains his style of writing.

Choice A is incorrect because that is just one single fact about the passage. Choice C is incorrect because that is just one single fact about the passage. Choice D is incorrect because that is just one single fact about the passage. Again, choice B is correct because it encompasses ALL the facts in the passage, not just one single fact.

**9. B**
The general tone is informal.

**10. B**
The statement, "Fewer people have aquariums in their office than at home," cannot be inferred from this article.

**11. C**
The author does not provide evidence for this statement.

**12. B**
The following statement is an opinion, " Aquarium gravel improves the aesthetics of the aquarium."

**13. A**
Secede means to break away from because the 11 states wanted to leave the United States and form their own country.

Choice B is incorrect because the states were not accomplishing anything. Choice C is incorrect because the states were trying to leave the USA not join it. Choice D is incorrect because the states seceded before they lost the war.

**14. B**
Look at the dates in the passage. The shots were fired on April 12 and Congress declared war on April 14.

Choice C is incorrect because the passage states that Lincoln was against slavery. Choice D is incorrect because it never mentions who was or was not at Fort Sumter.

**15. C**
The passage states that Lee surrendered to Grant after the capture of the capital of the Confederacy, which is Richmond.

Choice A is incorrect because the war continued for 2 years after Gettysburg. Choice B is incorrect because that battle is not mentioned in the passage. Choice D is incorrect because the capture of the capital occurred after the march to the sea.

**16. A**
**Truism:** n. self-evident or clear obvious truth.

**17. A**
**Virago:** Given to undue belligerence or ill manner at the slightest provocation; a shrew, a termagant.

**18. D**
**Femur:** n. The bone of the thigh or upper hind limb, articulating at the hip and the knee.

**19. C**
**Genteel:** Polite and well-mannered. Stylish or elegant. Aristocratic

**20. A**
**Adulterate:** v. To render (something) poorer in quality by adding another substance, typically an inferior one.

**21. B**
**Shrewd:** showing clever resourcefulness in practical matters, artful, tricky or cunning, streetwise, knowledgeable.

**22. A**
**Ulterior:** adj. beyond what is obvious or evident.

**23. B**
**Waif:** n. homeless child or stray.

**24. C**
**Princely:** adj. In the manner of a royal prince's conduct; large or grand.

**25. C**
**Deprecate:** v. To belittle or express disapproval of.

**26. D**
**Succor:** n. Aid, assistance or relief given to one in distress; ministration.

**27. B**
**Prominent:** adj. Important, famous.

**28. A**
**Alacrity:** adj. Eagerness; liveliness; enthusiasm.

**29. D**
**Cousins**

**30. C**
**Benevolent:** adj. Well meaning and kindly.

**31. B**
**Alleviate:** v. To make less severe, as a pain or difficulty.

**32. B**
**Benefactor:** n. Somebody who gives one a gift. Usually refers to someone who gives money to a charity or another form of organization.

**33. C**
**Underling:** n. Subordinate of lesser rank or authority.

**34. B**
**Specious:** adj. Seemingly well-reasoned or factual, but actually fallacious or insincere; strongly held but false.

**35. C**
**Proscribe:** v. To forbid or denounce.

**36. C**
**Veterinarian:** n. A person qualified to treat diseased or injured animals.

**37. C**
**Impeccable:** adj. Perfect, without faults, flaws or errors.

**38. A**
**Boisterous:** adj. Noisy, energetic, and cheerful; rowdy.

**39. B**
**Covert:** adj. Partially hidden, disguised, secret, surreptitious.

**40. B**
**Candid:** adj. Straightforward, open and sincere.

## Help with Reading Comprehension

At first sight, reading comprehension tests look challenging especially if you are given long essays to answer only two to three questions. While reading, you might notice your attention wandering, or feeling sleepy. Do not be discouraged because there are various tactics and long range strategies that make comprehending even long, boring essays easier.

**Your friends before your foes.** It is always best to start with essays or passages with familiar subjects rather than those with unfamiliar ones. This approach applies the same logic as tackling easy questions before hard ones. Skip passages that do not interest you and leave them for later.

Don't use 'special' reading techniques. This is not the time for speed-reading or anything like that – just plain ordinary reading – not too slow and not too fast.

**Read through the entire passage and the questions before you do anything.** Many students try reading the questions first and then looking for answers in the passage thinking this approach is more efficient. What these students do not realize is that it is often hard to navigate in unfamiliar roads. If you do not familiarize yourself with the passage first, looking for answers become not only time-consuming but also dangerous because you might miss the context of the answer you are looking for. If you read the questions first you will only confuse yourself and lose valuable time.

Familiarize yourself with reading comprehension questions. If you are familiar with the common types of reading comprehension questions, you are able to take note of important parts of the passage, saving time. There are six major kinds of reading comprehension questions.

- **Main Idea** - Questions that ask for the central thought or significance of the passage.

- **Specific Details** - Questions that asks for explicitly stated ideas.

- **Drawing Inferences** - Questions that ask for a statement's intended meaning.

- **Tone or Attitude** - Questions that test your ability to sense the emotional state of the author.

- **Context Meaning** – Questions that ask for the meaning of a word depending on the context.

- **Technique** – Questions that ask for the method of organization or the writing style of the author.

**Read. Read. Read**. The best preparation for reading comprehension tests is always to read, read and read. If you are not used to reading lengthy passages, you will probably lose concentration. Increase your attention span by making a habit out of reading.

Reading Comprehension tests become less daunting when you have trained yourself to read and understand fast. Always remember that it is easier to understand passages you are interested in. Do not read through passages hastily. Make mental notes of ideas you may be asked.

## Reading Comprehension Strategy

When facing the reading comprehension section of a standardized test, you need a strategy to be successful. You want to keep several steps in mind:

- First, make a note of the time and the number of sections. Time your work accordingly. Typically, four to five minutes per section is sufficient. Second, read the directions for each selection thoroughly before beginning (and listen well to any additional verbal instructions, as they will often clarify obscure or confusing written guidelines). You must know exactly how to do what you're about to do!

- Now you're ready to begin reading the selection. Read the passage carefully, noting significant characters or events on a scratch sheet of paper or underlining on the test sheet. Many students find making a basic list in the margins helpful. Quickly jot down or underline one-word summaries of characters, notable happenings, numbers, or key ideas. This will help you better retain information and focus wandering thoughts. Remember, however, that your main goal in doing this is to find the information that answers the questions. Even if you find the passage interesting, remember your goal and work fast but stay on track.

- Now read the question and all the choices. Now you have read the passage, have a general idea of the main ideas, and have marked the important points. Read the question and all the choices. Never choose an answer without reading them all! Questions are often designed to confuse – stay focussed and clear. Usually the answer choices will focus on one or two facts or inferences from the passage. Keep these clear in your mind.

- Search for the answer. With a very general idea of what the different choices are, go back to the passage and scan for the relevant information. Watch for big words, unusual or unique words. These make your job easier as you can scan the text for the particular word.

- Mark the Answer. Now you have the key information that the question is looking for. Go back to the question, quickly scan the choices and mark the correct one.

Understand and practice the different types of standardized reading comprehension tests. See the list above for the different types. Typically, there will be several questions dealing with facts from the selection, a couple more inference questions dealing with logical consequences of those facts, and periodically an application-oriented question surfaces to force you to make connections with what you already know. Some students prefer to answer the questions as listed, and feel classifying the question and then ordering is wasting precious time. Other students prefer to answer the different types of questions in order of how easy or difficult they are. The choice is yours and do whatever works for you. If you want to try answering in order of difficulty, here is a recommended order, answer fact questions first; they're easily found within the passage. Tackle inference problems next, after re-reading the question(s) as many times as you need to. Application or 'best guess' questions usually take the longest, so, save them for last.

Use the practice tests to try out both ways of answering and see what works for you.

For more help with reading comprehension, see Multiple Choice Secrets at www.multiple-choice.ca

## Main Idea, Topic and Supporting Details

Identifying the main idea, topic and supporting details in a passage can feel like an overwhelming task. The passages used for standardized tests can be boring and seem difficult. Test writers don't use interesting passages or ones that talk about things most people are familiar with. Despite these obstacles, all passages and paragraphs will have the information you need to answer the questions.

The topic of a passage or paragraph is its subject. It's the general idea and can be summed up in a word or short phrase. On some standardized tests, there is a short description of the passage if it's taken from a longer work. Make sure you read the description as it might state the topic of the passage. If not, read the passage and ask yourself, "Who or what is this about?" For example:

> Over the years, school uniforms have been hotly debated. Arguments are made that students have the right to show individuality and express themselves by choosing their own clothes. However, this brings up social and academic issues. Some kids cannot afford to wear the clothes they like and might be bullied by the "better dressed" students. With attention drawn to clothes and the individual, students will lose focus on class work and the reason they are in school. School uniforms should be mandatory.

**Ask:** What is this paragraph about?
**Topic:** school uniforms

Once you have the topic, it's easier to find the main idea. The main idea is a specific statement telling what the writer wants you to understand about the topic. Writers usually state the main idea as a thesis statement. If you're looking for the main idea of a single paragraph, the main idea is called the topic sentence and will probably be the first or last sentence. If you're looking for the main idea of an entire passage, look for the thesis statement in either the first or last paragraph. The main idea is usually restated in the conclusion. To find the main idea of a passage or paragraph, follow these steps:

1. Find the topic.

2. Ask yourself, "What point is the author trying to make about the topic?"

3. Create your own sentence summarizing the author's point.
4. Look in the text for the sentence closest in meaning to yours.

Look at the example paragraph again. It's already established that the topic of the paragraph is school uniforms. What is the main idea/topic sentence?

**Ask:** "What point is the author trying to make about school uniforms?"

**Summary:** Students should wear school uniforms.

**Topic sentence:** School uniforms should be mandatory.
**Main Idea:** School uniforms should be mandatory.

Each paragraph offers supporting details to explain the main idea. The details could be facts or reasons, but they will always answer a question about the main idea. What? Where? Why? When? How? How much/many? Look at the example paragraph again. You'll notice that more than one sentence answers a question about the main idea. These are the supporting details.

**Main Idea:** School uniforms should be mandatory.

**Ask:** Why?

> *Some kids cannot afford to wear clothes they like and could be bullied by the "better dressed" kids. **Supporting Detail**
>
> *With attention drawn to clothes and the individual, Students will lose focus on class work and the reason they are in school. **Supporting Detail**

What if the author doesn't state the main idea in a topic sentence? The passage will have an implied main idea. It's not as difficult to find as it might seem. Paragraphs are always organized around ideas. To find an implied main idea, you need to know the topic and then find the relationship between the supporting details. Ask yourself, "What is the point the author is making about the relationship between the details?"

> Cocoa is what makes chocolate good for you. Chocolate comes in many varieties. These delectable flavors include milk chocolate, dark chocolate, semi-sweet, and white chocolate.

**Ask:** What is this paragraph about?
**Topic:** Chocolate

**Ask:** What? Where? Why? When? How? How much/many?

**Supporting details:** Chocolate is good for you because it is made of cocoa, Chocolate is delicious, Chocolate comes in different delicious flavors

**Ask:** What is the relationship between the details and what is the author's point?

**Main Idea:** Chocolate is good because it is healthy and it tastes good.

## Testing Tips for Main Idea Questions

1. **Skim the questions** – not the answer choices - before reading the passage.

2. Questions about main idea might use the words "theme," "generalization," or "purpose."

3. **Save questions about the main idea for last.** Questions can often be found in order in the passage.

3. **Underline topic sentences in the passage.** Most tests allow you to write in your test booklet.

4. **Answer the question in your own words before looking at the answer choices.** Then match your answer with an answer choice.

5. **Cross out incorrect choices immediately to prevent confusion.**

6. **If two of the choices mean the same thing but use different words, they are BOTH incorrect.**

7. **If a question asks about the whole passage, cross out the choices that apply only to part of it.**

8. **If only part of the information is correct, that choice is incorrect.**

9. **An choice that is too broad is incorrect.** All information needs to be backed up by the passage.

10. **Choices with extreme wording are usually incorrect.**

## Reading Comprehension Strategy

When facing the reading comprehension section of a standardized test, you need a strategy to be successful. You want to keep several steps in mind:

- First, make a note of the time and the number of sections. Time your work accordingly. Typically, four to five minutes per section is sufficient. Second, read the directions for each selection thoroughly before beginning (and listen well to any additional verbal instructions, as they will often clarify obscure or confusing written guidelines). You must know exactly how to do what you're about to do!

- Now you're ready to begin reading the selection. Read the passage carefully, noting significant characters or events on a scratch sheet of paper or underlining on the test sheet. Many students find making a basic list in the margins helpful. Quickly jot down or underline one-word summaries of characters, notable happenings, numbers, or key ideas. This will help you better retain information and focus wandering thoughts. Remember, however, that your main goal in doing this is to find the information that answers the questions. Even if you find the passage interesting, remember your goal and work fast but stay on track.

- Now read the question and all the choices. Now you have read the passage, have a general idea of the main ideas, and have marked the important points. Read the question and all the choices. Never choose an answer without reading them all! Questions are often designed to confuse – stay focussed and clear. Usually the answer choices will focus on one or two facts or inferences from the passage. Keep these clear in your mind.

- Search for the answer. With a very general idea of what the different choices are, go back to the passage and scan for the relevant information. Watch for big words, unusual or unique words. These make your job easier as you can scan the text for the particular word.

- Mark the Answer. Now you have the key information that the question is looking for. Go back to the question, quickly scan the choices and mark the correct one.

Understand and practice the different types of standardized reading comprehension tests. See the list above for the different types. Typically, there will be several questions dealing with facts from the selection, a couple more inference questions dealing with logical consequences of those facts, and periodically an application-oriented question surfaces to force you to make connections with what you already know. Some students prefer to answer the questions as listed, and feel classifying the question and then ordering is wasting precious time. Other students prefer to answer the different types of questions in order of how easy or difficult they are. The choice is yours and do whatever works for you. If you want to try answering in order of difficulty, here is a recommended order, answer fact questions first; they're easily found within the passage. Tackle inference problems next, after re-reading the question(s) as many times as you need to. Application or 'best guess' questions usually take the longest, so, save them for last.

Use the practice tests to try out both ways of answering and see what works for you.

For more help with reading comprehension, see Multiple Choice Secrets at www.multiple-choice.ca.

## Drawing Inferences And Conclusions

Drawing inferences and making conclusions happens all the time. In fact, you probably do it every time you read—sometimes without even realizing it! For example, remember the first time you saw the movie "The Lion King." When you meet Scar for the first time, he is trapping a helpless mouse with his sharp claws preparing to eat it. When you see this action you guess that Scar is going to be a bad character in the movie. Nothing appeared to tell you this. No caption came across the bottom of the screen that said "Bad Guy." No red arrow pointed to Scar and said "Evil Lion." No, you made an inference about his character based on the context clue you were given. You do the same thing when you read!

When you draw an inference or make a conclusion you are doing the same thing, you are making an educated guess based on the hints the author gives you. We call these hints "context clues." Scar trapping the innocent mouse is the context clue about Scar's character.

Usually you are making inferences and drawing conclusions the entire time you are reading. Whether you realize it or not, you are constantly making educated guesses based on context clues. Think about a time you were reading a book and something happened that you were expecting to happen. You're not psychic! Actually, you were picking up on the context clues and making inferences about what was going to happen next!

Let's try an easy example. Read the following sentences and answer the questions at the end of the passage.

> Shelly really likes to help people. She loves her job because she gets to help people every single day. However, Shelly has to work long hours and she can get called in the middle of the night for emergencies. She wears a white lab coat at work and usually she carries a stethoscope.

**What is Shelly's job?**

   a. Musician
   b. Lawyer
   c. Doctor
   d. Teacher


This probably seemed easy. Drawing inferences isn't always this simple, but it is the same basic principle. How did you know Shelly was a doctor? She helps people, she works long hours, she wears a white lab coat, and she gets called in for emergencies at night. Context Clues! Nowhere in the paragraph did it say Shelly was a doctor, but you were able to draw that conclusion based on the information provided in the paragraph. This is how it's done!

There is a catch, though. Remember that when you draw inferences based on reading, you should only use the information given to you by the author. Sometimes it is easy for us to make conclusions based on knowledge that is already in our mind—but that can lead you to drawing an incorrect inference. For example, let's pretend there is a bully at your school named Brent. Now let's say you read a story and the main character's name is Brent. You could NOT infer that the character in the story is a bully just because his name is Brent. You should only use the information given to you by the author to avoid drawing the wrong conclusion.

Let's try another example.

> Social media is an extremely popular new form of connecting and communicating over the internet. Since Facebook's original launch in 2004, millions of people have joined in the social media craze. In fact, it is estimated that almost 75% of all internet users aged 18 and older use some form of social media. Facebook started at Harvard University as a way to get students connected. However, it quickly grew into a worldwide phenomenon and today, the founder of Facebook, Mark Zuckerberg has an estimated net worth of 28.5 billion dollars.
>
> Facebook is not the only social media platform, though. Other sites such as Twitter, Instagram, and Snapchat have since been invented and are quickly becoming just as popular! Many social media users actually use more than one type of social media. Furthermore, most social media sites have created mobile apps that allow people to connect via social media virtually anywhere in the world!

What is the most likely reason that other social media sites like Twitter and Instagram were created?

> a. Professors at Harvard University made it a class project.
>
> b. Facebook was extremely popular and other people thought they could also be successful by designing social media sites.
>
> c. Facebook was not connecting enough people.
>
> d. Mark Zuckerberg paid people to invent new social media sites because he wanted lots of competition.

Here, the correct answer is B. Facebook was extremely popular and other people thought they could also be successful by designing social media sites. How do we know this? What are the context clues? Take a look at the first paragraph. What do we know based on this paragraph? Well, one sentence refers to Facebook's original launch. This suggests that Facebook was one of the first social media sites. In addition, we know that the founder of Facebook has been extremely successful and is worth billions of dollars. From this we can infer that other people wanted to imitate Facebook's idea and become just as successful as Mark Zuckerberg.

Let's go through the other answers. If you chose A, it might be because Facebook started at Harvard University, so you drew the conclusion that all other social media sites were also started at Harvard University. However, there is no mention of class projects, professors, or students designing social media. So there doesn't seem to be enough support for choice A.

If you chose C, you might have been drawing your own conclusions based on outside information. Maybe none of your friends are on Facebook, so you made an inference that Facebook didn't connect enough people, so more sites were invented. Or maybe you think the people who connect on Facebook are too old, so you don't think Facebook connects enough people your age. This might be true, but remember inferences should be drawn from the information the author gives you!

If you chose D, you might be using the information that Mark Zuckerberg is worth over 28 billion dollars. It would be easy for him to pay others to design new sites, but remember, you need to use context clues! He is very wealthy, but that statement was giving you information about how successful Facebook was—not suggesting that he paid others to design more sites!

So remember, drawing inferences and conclusions is simply about using the information you are given to make an educated guess. You do this every single day so don't let this concept scare you. Look for the context clues, make sure they support your claim, and you'll be able to make accurate inferences and conclusions!

## Meaning From Context

Often in Reading Comprehension questions, you are asked for the definition of a word, which you have to infer from the surrounding text, called "meaning in context." Here are a few examples with step-by-step solutions, and a few tips and tricks to answering meaning from context questions.

There are literally thousands and thousands of words in the English language. It is impossible for us to know what every single one of them means, but we also don't have time to Google a definition every time we read a word we don't understand! Even the smartest person in the world comes across words they don't know, but luckily we can use context clues to help us determine what things actually mean.

Context clues are really just little hints that can help us determine the meaning of words or phrases and honestly, the easiest way to learn how to use context clues is to practice!

Let's start with a few basic examples.

> In some countries many people are not given access to schools, teachers, or books. In these countries, people might be illiterate.

You might not know what the word illiterate means, but let's use the clues in the sentence to help us. If people are not given access to schools, teachers, or books, what might happen? They probably don't learn what we learned in school so they might not know some of the things that we learned from our teachers! Illiterate actually means "unable to read or write." This makes sense based on the context clues!

Let's work through another example.

> We have so much technology today! So much technology that many people have started using tablets and computers to read ebooks instead of paper books! In fact, some of these people actually think that reading paper books is archaic!

Let's look for the context clues. Well, what do we know from this paragraph? We have a lot of technology and sometimes people read ebooks instead of paper books. From this we can draw the conclusion that ebooks are beginning to replace paper books because ebooks are newer and better. So if ebooks are newer and better, it must mean that paper books are older. Archaic actually means "very old or old-fashioned," which again we determined from the context clues.

Let's see if you can try a few on your own now.

> Cody noticed the strawberries in his refrigerator were old and moldy, so he abstained and threw them away. What does abstained most likely mean?
> 
> a. chose not to consume
> b. washed
> c. shared
> d. cut into pieces

The correct answer here is A. The context clues told you the strawberries were old and moldy and also told you that Cody did something and then threw them away. If the strawberries were moldy, and Cody abstained, it makes sense that he didn't eat them—which is choice A.

You may have chosen answer B. If the strawberries were old and moldy, Cody could have washed them. But use ALL of the context clues. After he abstained, he threw them away. Why would Cody wash them and then throw them away? That doesn't make sense! In addition, why would he share them if they were old and moldy? Finally, I suppose Cody could have cut them into pieces, but why would he need to do that before throwing them away? It doesn't make as much sense, so choice A is the correct answer!

Let's do one more.

> Scott had a disdain for Lily ever since she lied to their boss and got him fired.
> 
> a. Compassion
> b. Hate
> c. Remorse
> d. Money

The correct answer is B. Scott was fired because Lily lied. Can you imagine if this happened to you? I think you would have some pretty strong feelings just like Scott!

It's simple! By understanding the context, you can determine the meaning of even the hardest of words!

## Help with Building your Vocabulary

Vocabulary tests can be daunting when you think of the enormous number of words that might come up in the exam. As the exam date draws near, your anxiety will grow because you know that no matter how many words you memorize, chances are, you will still remember so few. Here are some tips which you can use to hurdle the big words that may come up in your exam without having to open the dictionary and memorize all the words known to humankind.
How to memorize
https://www.test-preparation.ca/a-guide-to-memorizing-anything-easily-and-painlessly/
Build up and tear apart the big words. Big words, like many other things, are composed of small parts. Some words are made up of many other words. A man who lifts weights for example, is a weight lifter. Words are also made up of parts called prefixes, suffixes and roots. Often times, we can see the relationship of different words through these parts. A person who is skilled with both hands is ambidextrous. A word with double meaning is ambiguous. A person with two conflicting emotions is ambivalent. Two words with synonymous meanings often have the same root. Bio, a root word derived from Latin is used in words like biography meaning to write about a person's life, and biology meaning the study of living organisms.

- **Words with double meanings.** Did you know that the word husband not only means a man married to a woman, but also thrift or frugality? Sometimes, words have double meanings. The dictionary meaning, or the denotation of a word is sometimes different from the way we use it or its connotation.

- **Read widely, read deeply and read daily.** The best way to expand your vocabulary is to familiarize yourself with as many words as possible through reading. By reading, you are able to remember words in a proper context and thus, remember its meaning or at the very least, its use. Reading widely would help you get acquainted with words you may never use every day. This is the best strategy without doubt. However, if you are studying for an exam next week, or even tomorrow, it isn't much help! Below you will find a range of different ways to learn new words quickly and efficiently.

- **Remember.** Always remember that big words are easy to understand when divided into smaller parts, and the smaller words will often have several other meanings aside from the one you already know.

Here are suggested effective ways to help you improve your vocabulary.

**Be Committed To Learning New Words**. To improve your vocabulary you need to make a commitment to learn new words. Commit to learning at least a word or two a day. You can also get new words by reading books, poems, stories, plays and magazines. Expose yourself to more language to increase the number of new words that you learn.

- **Learn Practical Vocabulary**. As much as possible, learn vocabulary that is associated with what you do and that you can use regularly. For example learn words related to your profession or hobby. Learn as much vocabulary as you can in your favorite subjects.

- **Use New Words Frequently**. When you learn a new word start using it and do so frequently. Repeat it when you are alone and try to use the word as often as you can with people you talk to. You can also use flashcards to practice new words that you learn.

- **Learn the Proper Usage.** If you do not understand the proper usage, look it up and make sure you have it right.

- **Use a Dictionary**. When reading textbooks, novels or assigned readings, keep the dictionary nearby. Also learn how to use online dictionaries and WORD dictionary. When you come across a new word, check for its meaning. If you cannot do so immediately, then you should write it down and check it when possible. This will help you understand what the word means and exactly how best to use it.

- **Learn Word Roots, Prefixes and Suffixes.** English words are usually derived from suffixes, prefixes and roots, which come from Latin, French or Greek. Learning the root or origin of a word helps you easily understand the meaning of the word and other words that are derived from the root. Generally, if you learn the meaning of one root word, you will understand two or three words. This is a great two-for-one strategy. Most prefixes, suffixes, roots and stems are used in two, three or more words, so if you know the root, prefix or suffix, you can guess the meaning of many words.

- **Synonyms and Antonyms**. Most words in the English language have two or three (at least) synonyms and antonyms. For example, "big," in the most common usage, has about seventy-five synonyms and an equal number of antonyms. Understanding the relationships between these words and how they all fit together gives your brain a framework, which makes them easier to learn, remember and recall.

- **Use Flash Cards**. Flash cards are the best way to memorize things. They can be used anywhere and anytime, so you can use free moments waiting for the bus or waiting in line. Make your own or buy commercially prepared flash cards, and keep them with you all the time. See https://www.test-preparation.ca/test-preparation-with-flash-cards/

- **Make word lists.** Learning vocabulary, like learning many things, requires repetition. Keep a new words journal in a separate section or separate notebook. Add any words that you look up in the dictionary, as well as from word lists. Review your word lists regularly.

Photocopying or printing off word lists from the Internet or handouts is not the same. Actually writing out the word and a few notes on the definition is an important process for imprinting the word in your brain. Writing out the word and definition in your New Word Journal, forces you to concentrate and focus on the new word. Hitting PRINT or pushing the button on the photocopier does not do the same thing.

Notice the verbs in bold in the examples above. They are encircling the subjects of each sentence rather than following them. This is inverse word order.

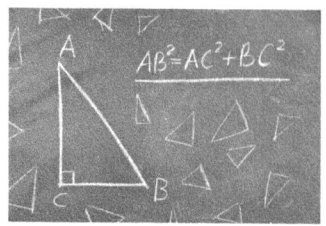

# MATHEMATICS

THIS SECTION CONTAINS A SELF-ASSESSMENT AND MATH TUTORIALS. The Tutorials are designed to familiarize general principles and the self-assessment contains general questions similar to the reading questions likely to be on the PAX RN exam, but are not intended to be identical to the exam questions. Many Universities recommend that students take introductory courses before taking the PAX RN Exam. The tutorials are not designed to be a complete mathematics course, and it is assumed that students have some familiarity with math questions. If you do not understand parts of the tutorial, or find the tutorial difficult, it is recommended that you seek out additional instruction.

## Tour of the PAX RN Mathematics Content

The PAX RN reading section has 50 questions. Below is a more detailed list of the types of math questions that generally appear on the PAX RN.

- Basic operations - adding, subtracting, multiplying and dividing whole numbers
- Square root
- Prime factors
- Median and mode
- Exponents
- Word problems
- Simple geometry
- IQ questions
- Operations with polynomials
- Quadratics
- Ratio and proportion

- Fractions, decimals and percent
- Speed, acceleration and momentum

The questions below are not the same as you will find on the PAX RN - that would be too easy! And nobody knows what the questions will be and they change all the time. Mostly the changes consist of substituting new questions for old, but the changes can be new question formats or styles, changes to the number of questions in each section, changes to the time limits for each section and combining sections. Below are general math questions that cover the same areas as the PAX RN. So the format and exact wording of the questions may differ slightly, and change from year to year, if you can answer the questions below, you will have no problem with the math section of the PAX RN.

## Math Self-Assessment

The purpose of the self-assessment is:

- Identify your strengths and weaknesses.
- Develop your personalized study plan (above)
- Get accustomed to the PAX RN format
- Extra practice – the self-assessments are almost a full 3rd practice test!
- Provide a baseline score for preparing your study schedule.

Since this is a Self-assessment, and depending on how confident you are with math, timing is optional. The PAX RN has 50 reading questions to be answered in 50 minutes. The self-assessment has 50 questions, so allow 50 minutes to complete this assessment.

Once complete, use the table below to assess your understanding of the content, and prepare your study schedule described in chapter 1.

| 80% - 100%    | Excellent – you have mastered the content                                                                                                                                                |
| ------------- | ---------------------------------------------------------------------------------------------------------------------------------------------------------------------------------------- |
| 60 – 79%      | Good. You have a working knowledge. Even though you can just pass this section, you may want to review the tutorials and do some extra practice to see if you can improve your mark.     |
| 40% - 59%     | Below Average. You do not understand the math problems. Review the tutorials, and retake this quiz again in a few days, before proceeding to the rest of the Practice Test.              |
| Less than 40% | Poor. You have a very limited understanding of math. Please review the tutorials, and retake this quiz again in a few days, before proceeding to the rest of the study guide.            |

**Math Self-Assessment Answer Sheet**

1. A B C D
2. A B C D
3. A B C D
4. A B C D
5. A B C D
6. A B C D
7. A B C D
8. A B C D
9. A B C D
10. A B C D
11. A B C D
12. A B C D
13. A B C D
14. A B C D
15. A B C D
16. A B C D
17. A B C D
18. A B C D
19. A B C D
20. A B C D
21. A B C D
22. A B C D
23. A B C D
24. A B C D
25. A B C D
26. A B C D
27. A B C D
28. A B C D
29. A B C D
30. A B C D
31. A B C D
32. A B C D
33. A B C D
34. A B C D
35. A B C D
36. A B C D
37. A B C D
38. A B C D
39. A B C D
40. A B C D
41. A B C D
42. A B C D
43. A B C D
44. A B C D
45. A B C D
46. A B C D
47. A B C D
48. A B C D
49. A B C D
50. A B C D

# Mathematics Self-Assessment

## Decimals, Fractions and Percent

1. A person earns $25000 per month and pays $9000 income tax per year. The Government increased income tax by 0.5% per month and his monthly earning was raised $11000. How much more income tax does he pay per month?

   a. $1260
   b. $1050
   c. $750
   d. $510

2. A boy has 5 red balls, 3 white balls and 2 yellow balls. What percent of the balls are yellow?

   a. 2%
   b. 8%
   c. 20%
   d. 12%

3. There were some oranges in a basket, by adding 8/5 of these, the total became 130. How many oranges were in the basket?

   a. 60
   b. 50
   c. 40
   d. 35

4. A 7 centimeter diameter pizza weighs 750 grams. If the diameter increased to 8.2 centimeters, how much more will it weigh?

   a. 279
   b. 129
   c. 185
   d. 305

5. A distributor purchased 550 kilograms of potatoes for $165. He distributed these at a rate of $6.4 per 20 kilograms to 15 shops, $3.4 per 10 kilograms to 12 shops and the remainder at $1.8 per 5 kilograms. If his total distribution cost is $10, what will his profit be?

   a. $10.40
   b. $8.60
   c. $14.90
   d. $23.40

6. Convert 0.45 to a fraction

   a. 7/20
   b. 7/45
   c. 9/20
   d. 3/20

7. How much pay does Mr. Johnson receive if he gives half of his pay to his family, $250 to his landlord, and has exactly 3/7 of his pay left after these expenses?

   a. $3600
   b. $3500
   c. $2800
   d. $1750

**8. What is the square root of √225?**

   a. 25
   b. 15
   c. 5
   d. 13

**9. A man buys an item for $420 and has a balance of 3000.00. How much did he have before?**

   a. $2,580
   b. $3,420
   c. $2,420
   d. $342

**10. Divide 9.60 by 3.2**

   a. 2.50
   b. 3
   c. 2.3
   d. 6.4

**11. If a discount of 20% is given for a desk and Mark saves $45, how much did he pay for the desk?**

   a. $225
   b. $160
   c. $180
   d. $210

**12. 10% of p is also 1/5 of q. Which of the following is correct?**

   a. p + p = q
   b. q/p = p
   c. p - q = q
   d. p/q = p

## Basic Algebra

**13. If X = 7 solve 3x + 5 − 2x**

   a. x = 6
   b. x = 12
   c. x = 1
   d. x = 0

**14. Solve the following equation 3(2x − 2) = 24 − 3x**

   a. x = 24
   b. x = 9
   c. x = 10
   d. x = 3.33

**15. Expand (x + 7) (x - 3)**

   a. $x^2$ + 4x − 21
   b. x + 21
   c. 2x + 4 − 21
   d. 6x - 21

## Mean Mode and Median

**16. Find the mean of 100, 1050, 320, 600 and 150.**

   a. 333
   b. 444
   c. 440
   d. 320

**17. Find the median of the set of numbers – 1,2,3,4,5,6,7,8,9 and 10.**

    a. 55
    b. 10
    c. 1
    d. 5.5

**18. The following represents the age distribution of students in an elementary class. Find the mode of the values – 7, 9, 10, 13, 11, 7, 9, 19, 12, 11, 9, 7, 9, 10, 11**

    a. 7
    b. 9
    c. 10
    d. 11

## Exponents

**19. Express in $3^4$ standard form**

    a. 81
    b. 27
    c. 12
    d. 9

**20. Simplify $4^3 + 2^4$**

    a. 45
    b. 108
    c. 80
    d. 48

**21. If x = 2 and y = 5, solve $xy^3 - x^3$**

    a. 240
    b. 258
    c. 248
    d. 242

**22. $X^3 \times X^2 =$**

    a. $5^x$
    b. $x^{-5}$
    c. $x^{-1}$
    d. $x^5$

**23. Express $100000^0$ in standard form.**

    a. 1
    b. 0
    c. 100000
    d. 1000

**24. Solve $\sqrt{144}$**

    a. 14
    b. 72
    c. 24
    d. 12

# Geometry

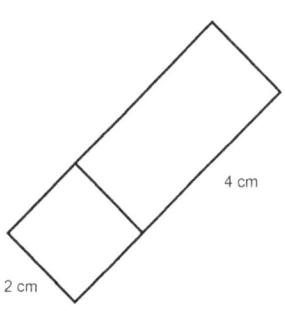

Note: Figure not drawn to scale

**25. Assuming the shape with a 2 cm. side is square, what is perimeter of the above shape?**

a. 12 cm
b. 16 cm
c. 6 cm
d. 20 cm

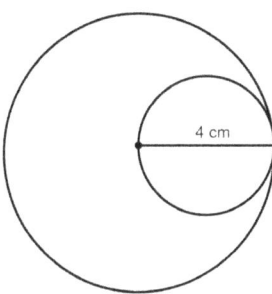

Note: Figure not drawn to scale

**26. Assuming the diameter of the radius of the larger circle, what is (area of large circle) - (area of small circle) in the figure above?**

a. 8 π cm²
b. 10 π cm²
c. 12 π cm²
d. 16 π cm²

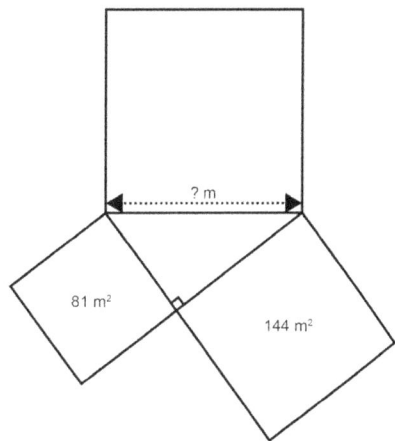

Note: Figure not drawn to scale

**27. Assuming all 3 shapes around the center right-triangle are square, what is the length of each side of the square above?**

a. 10
b. 15
c. 20
d. 5

**28. A bag contains 38 black balls and 42 white balls. What is the ratio of black balls to white?**

a. 9:11
b. 1:3
c. 19:21
d. 11:9

**29. The ratio of 8:5 = (?)%**

a. 75%
b. 150%
c. 175%
d. 160%

**30.** 3 boys are asked to clean a surface that is 4 ft². If the portion is divided equally among the boys, what size will each of them clean?

   a. 1 ft 6 inches²
   b. 14 inches²
   c. 1 ft 2 inches²
   d. 1 ft² 48 inches²

**31.** Brian jogged 7 times around a circular track 75 meters in diameter. How much linear distance did he cover?

   a. 1250 meters
   b. 1650 meters
   c. 1450 meters
   d. 1725 meters

**32.** Consider the following population growth chart.

| Country | Population 2000 | Population 2005 |
|---|---|---|
| Japan | 122,251,000 | 128,057,000 |
| China | 1,145,195,000 | 1,341,335,000 |
| United States | 253,339,000 | 310,384,000 |
| Indonesia | 184,346,000 | 239,871,000 |

Which country is growing the fastest?

   a. Japan
   b. China
   c. United States
   d. Indonesia

## Basic Math

**33.** $467 \times 41 =$

   a. 19,147
   b. 21,227
   c. 23,107
   d. 18,177

**34.** $1518 \div 27 =$

   a. 54 r1
   b. 56 r6
   c. 55 r3
   d. 59 r2

**35.** $7050 - 305 =$

   a. 6705
   b. 6745
   c. 5745
   d. 6045

**36.** $8327 - 1278 =$

   a. 7149
   b. 7209
   c. 6059
   d. 7049

**37.** $285 \times 12 =$

   a. 3420
   b. 3402
   c. 3024
   d. 2322

38. 46 × 15 =

   a. 590
   b. 690
   c. 490
   d. 790

39. 5575 + 8791 =

   a. 14,756
   b. 14,566
   c. 14,466
   d. 14,366

40. What are the prime factors of 17?

   a. 2 x 8.5
   b. 17
   c. 3 x 5.5
   d. None of the above

41. What are the prime factors of 100?

   a. 2 x 2 x 5 x 5
   b. 4 x 25
   c. 2 x 2 x 2 x 5 x 5
   d. 2 x 50

## Speed and Momentum

42. Three cars are travelling down an even road at a velocity of 110 m/s, calculate the car with the highest momentum if they are all moving at the same speed, but the first car weighs 2500 kg, second car weighs 2650 kg and third car weighs 2009 kg?

   a. First car
   b. Second car
   c. Third car
   d. All have same momentum

43. What is the momentum of a log of wood that weighs 700 kg rolling down a hill at 4.6 m/s?

   a. 3220 kg x m/s down hill
   b. 3320 kg x m/s
   c. 3320 down hill
   d. 3320 M

## Quadratics and Polynomials

44. It is known that $x^2 + 4x = 5$. Then x can be

   a. 0
   b. -5
   c. 1
   d. Either (b) or (c)

45. Add $-3x^2 + 2x + 6$ and $-x^2 - x - 1$.

   a. $-2x^2 + x + 5$
   b. $-4x^2 + x + 5$
   c. $-2x^2 + 3x + 5$
   d. $-4x^2 + 3x + 5$

46. Simplify the following expression:

$3x^3 + 2x^2 + 5x - 7 + 4x^2 - 5x + 2 - 3x^3$

   a. $6x^2 - 9$
   b. $6x^2 - 5$
   c. $6x^2 - 10x - 5$
   d. $6x^2 + 10x - 9$

## Scientific Notation

**47. Convert 7,892,000,000 to scientific notation**

  a. $7.892 \times 10^{10}$
  b. $7.892 \times 10^{-9}$
  c. $7.892 \times 10^{9}$
  d. $0.7892 \times 10^{11}$

**48. Convert 0.045 to scientific notation**

  a. $4.5 \times 10^{-2}$
  b. $4.5 \times 10^{2}$
  c. $4.05 \times 10^{-2}$
  d. $4.5 \times 10^{-3}$

## Non-verbal IQ

**Select the figure with the same relationship.**

49.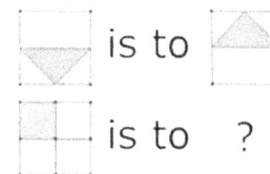

50. □ is to ⌐¬

    ⬠ is to ?

    a. ⌒   b. ◠

    c. ⌃   d. ⊔

## Answer Key

## Decimals, Percent and Fractions

**1. D**
With the new tax rate, income tax is 3.5%. Per month income tax = $9000/12 = $750. Per month income tax rate = $750 X 100/$25,000 = 3%. Income per month = $25,000 + $11,000 = $36,000. Monthly tax amount = $36,000 X 0.035 = $1260. Amount of additional tax = $1260 - $750 = $510

**2. C**
Total no. of balls = 10, no. of yellow balls = 2, answer = 2/10 X 100 = 20%

**3. B**
Suppose oranges in the basket before = x, Then: X + 8x/5 = 130, 5x + 8x = 650, so X = 50.

**4. A**
The area of a 7 centimeter pizza is $\prod(3.5)^2$ × = 38.48 cm². The weight of 1 cm² of pizza will be 750/38.48 = 19.49 grams. The area of a 8.2 centimeter diameter pizza is $\prod (4.1)^2$ = 52.81 cm². The difference in area is 52.81 – 38.48 = 14.33 cm². The difference in weight will be 19.49 X 14.33 = 279.29 grams.

**5. B**
The distribution is done in three different rates and amounts:

$6.4 per 20 kilograms to 15 shops ... 20 * 15 = 300 kilograms distributed

$3.4 per 10 kilograms to 12 shops ... 10 * 12 = 120 kilograms distributed

550 - (300 + 120) = 550 - 420 = 130 kilograms left. This amount is distributed in 5 kilogram portions. So, this means that there are 130/5 = 26 shops.

$1.8 per 130 kilograms.

We need to find the amount he earned overall these distributions.

$6.4 per 20 kilograms : 6.4 * 15 = $96 for 300 kilograms

$3.4 per 10 kilograms : 3.4 * 12 = $40.8 for 120 kilograms

$1.8 per 5 kilograms : 1.8 * 26 = $46.8 for 130 kilograms

So, he earned 96 + 40.8 + 46.8 = $ 183.6

The total cost of distribution is given as $10

The profit is found by: Money earned - money spent ... It is important to remember that he bought 550 kilograms of potatoes for $165 at the beginning:

Profit = 183.6 - 10 - 165 = $8.6

**6. C**
0.45 = 45/100 = 9/20

**7. B**
We check the fractions taking place in the question. We see that there is a "half" (that is 1/2) and 3/7. So, we multiply the denominators of these fractions to decide how to name the total money. We say that Mr. Johnson has 14x at the beginning; he gives half of this, meaning 7x, to his family. $250 to his landlord. He has 3/7 of his money left. 3/7 of 14x is equal to:

14x * (3/7) = 6x

So,

Spent money is: 7x + 250

Unspent money is: 6x

Total money is: 14x

We write an equation: total money = spent

money + unspent money

14x = 7x + 250 + 6x

14x - 7x - 6x = 250

x = 250

We are asked to find the total money that is 14x:

14x = 14 * 250 = $3500

**8. B**
$\sqrt{225}$ = 15.

**9. B**
(Amount Spent) $420 + $3000 (Balance) = $3420

**10. B**
9.60/3.2 = 3

**11. C**
By the given information in the question, we understand that the discounted part is the saved amount. If we say that the original price of the desk is 100x; by 20% discount rate, 20x will be the discounted part:

20x = 45

We know that Mark paid 20% less than the original price. So, he paid 100x - 20x = 80x. We are asked to find 80x. With a simple direct proportion, we can find the result:

20x = 45

80x = ?

By cross multiplication, we find the result:

? = 80x•45 / 20x = 4•45 = $180

**12. C**
First convert to percent. 1/5 = 20%, so 10% of p = 20% of q, and p = 2 X q, and p - q = q

## Basic Algebra

**13. B**
X = 7, so 3x = 3 x 7 = 21, 2x = 2 x 7 = 14, so 21 + 5 - 14 = 26 - 14 = 12

**14. D**
6x – 6 = 24 – 3x
6x + 3x - 6 = 24
9x – 6 = 24
9x = 24 + 6
9x = 30
x = 30/9
x = 3.33

**15. A**
Multiply the first bracket and the second.
$x^2$ - 3x + 7x - 21 = $x^2$ + 4x – 21

## Mean and Mode

**16. B**
First add all the numbers 100 + 1050 + 320 + 600 + 150 = 2220. Then divide by 5 (the number of data provided) = 2220/5 = 444

**17. D**
First arrange the numbers in a numerical sequence - 1,2,3,4,5,6,7,8,9, 10. Then find the middle number or numbers. The middle numbers are 5 and 6. The median = 5 + 6/2 = 11/2 = 5.5

**18. B**
Find the most recurring number. The most occurring number in the series is 9

## Exponents

**19. A**
3 x 3 x 3 x 3 = 81

**20. C**
(4 x 4 x 4) + (2 x 2 x 2 x 2) = 64 + 16 = 80

**21. D**
$2(5)^3 - (2)^3 = 2(125) - 8 = 250 - 8 = 242$

**22. D**
$X^3 \times X^2 = X^{3+2} = X^5$
To multiply exponents with like bases, add the exponents.

**23. A**
Any value (except 0) raised to the power of 0 equals 1.

**24. D**
$\sqrt{144} = 12$

## Geometry

**25. B**
We see that there is a square with side 2 cm. and a rectangle adjacent to it, with one side 2 cm. (common side with the square) and the other side 4 cm. The perimeter of a shape is found by summing up all sides surrounding the shape, not adding the ones inside the shape. Three 2 cm sides from the square, and two 4 cm sides and one 2 cm side from the rectangle contribute the perimeter.

So, the perimeter of the shape is: 2 + 2 + 2 + 4 + 2 + 4 = 16 cm.

**26. C**
In the figure, we are given a large circle and a small circle inside it; with the diameter equal to the radius of the large one. The diameter of the small circle is 4 cm. This means that its radius is 2 cm. Since the diameter of the small circle is the radius of the large circle, the radius of the large circle is 4 cm. The area of a circle is calculated by: $πr^2$ where r is the radius.

Area of the small circle: $π(2)^2 = 4π$

Area of the large circle: $π(4)^2 = 16π$

The difference area is found by:

Area of the large circle - Area of the small circle = $16π - 4π = 12π$

**27. B**
We see that there are three squares forming a right triangle in the middle. Two of the squares have the areas 81 m² and 144 m². If we denote their sides a and b respectively:

$a^2 = 81$ and $b^2 = 144$. The length which is asked is the hypotenuse; a and b are the opposite and adjacent sides of the right angle. By using the Pythagorean Theorem, we can find the value of the asked side:

**Pythagorean Theorem:**

$(Hypotenuse)^2 = (Opposite\ Side)^2 + (Adjacent\ Side)^2$

$h^2 = a^2 + b^2$

$a^2 = 81$ and $b^2 = 144$ are given. So;

$h^2 = 81 + 144$

$h^2 = 225$

$h = 15$ m

**28. C**
The ratio of black balls to white is 38:42. Reduce to lowest terms = 19:21

**29. D**
The ratio 8:5 = X/100
X = 160%

**30. D**
1 foot is equal to 12 inches. So 1 ft² = 12 * 12 in²

4 ft² = 4 * 12 * 12 in² = 576 in²

The surface area is divided equally among 3 boys.

Each boy will clean 576/3 = 192 in²

192 in² = 144 in² + 48 in²; 144 in² = 1 ft²

So, each boy will clean 1 ft² and 48 in²

**31. B**
In one round-trip, he covers the circumference of the path. 75/X = 3.14159. 75 X 3.14159 = X. Circumference of the path = X = 235.65 meters. Distance covered 7 times around = 235.65 × 7 = 1650 meters.

**32. D**
Indonesia is growing the fastest at about 30%.

**33. A**
467 × 41 = 19,147

**34. B**
1518 ÷ 27 = 56 r6

**35. B**
7050 − 305 = 6745

**36. D**
8327 − 1278 = 7049

**37. A**
285 × 12 = 3420

**38. B**
46 × 15 = 690

**39. D**
5575 + 8791 = 14366

**40. B**
The only prime number that can divide 17 is 17.

**41. A**
To make it easier we can break this large number to two smaller numbers, 2 x 50 or 4 x 25. Let's use 4 x 25. The prime factors of 4 = 2 x 2, and the prime factors of 25 = 5 x 5. The prime factors of 100 = 2 x 2 x 5 x 5

**42. C**
Momentum is a product of velocity and mass. If they are all travelling at the same speed, the car that weighs the most (the second car) would have the highest momentum.

**43. A**
The momentum of a log of wood that weighs 700kg rolling down a hill at 4.6m/s will be 4.6 X 700 = 3220 kg x m/s down hill.

## Quadratics and Polynomials

**44. D**
$x^2 + 4x = 5$, $x^2 + 4x - 5 = 0$, $x^2 + 5x - x - 5 = 0$, factoring $x(x + 5) - 1(x + 5) = 0$, $(x + 5)(x-1)=0$. $x + 5 = 0$ or $x - 1 = 0$, $x = 0 - 5$ or $x = 0 + 1$, $x = -5$ or $x = 1$, either b or c.

**45. B**
$(-3x^2 + 2x + 6) + (-x^2 - x - 1)$

$= -3x^2 + 2x + 6 - x^2 - x - 1$ ... we write similar terms together:

$= -3x^2 - x^2 + 2x - x + 6 - 1$ ... we operate within the same terms:

$= -4x^2 + x + 5$

**46. B**
$3x^3 + 2x^2 + 5x - 7 + 4x^2 - 5x + 2 - 3x^3$ ... we write similar terms together:
$= 3x^3 - 3x^3 + 2x^2 + 4x^2 + 5x - 5x - 7 + 2$ ... we operate within the same terms. $3x^3$ and $-3x^3$, $5x$ and $-5x$ cancel:

$= 6x^2 - 5$

## Scientific Notation

**47. C**
The decimal point moves 9 spaces right to be placed after 7, which is the first non-zero number. Thus $7.892 \times 10^9$

**48. A**
The decimal point moves 2 spaces to the left to be placed before 4, which is the

first non-zero number. Thus its $4.5 \times 10^{-2}$
The answer is negative since the decimal moved left.

## Non-verbal IQ

**49. D**
The relationship is the same figure flipped vertically, so the best choice is D.

**50. C**
The relation is the same figure with the bottom half removed.

## Basic Math Video Tutorials

https://www.test-preparation.ca/basic-math-video-tutorials/

## Fraction Tips, Tricks and Shortcuts

When you are writing an exam, time is precious, and anything you can do to answer questions faster, is a real advantage. Here are some ideas, shortcuts, tips and tricks that can speed up answering fraction problems.

Remember that a fraction is just a number which names a portion of something. For instance, instead of having a whole pie, a fraction says you have a part of a pie--such as a half of one or a fourth of one.

Two digits make up a fraction. The digit on top is known as the numerator. The digit on the bottom is known as the denominator. To remember which is which, just remember that "denominator" and "down" both start with a "d." And the "downstairs" number is the denominator. So for instance, in ½, the numerator is the 1 and the denominator (or "downstairs") number is the 2.

- It's easy to add two fractions if they have the same denominator. Just add the digits on top and leave the bottom one the same: 1/10 + 6/10 = 7/10.

- It's the same with subtracting fractions with the same denominator: 7/10 - 6/10 = 1/10.

- Adding and subtracting fractions with different denominators is more complicated. First, you have to get the problem so that they do have the same denominators. One easiest way to do this is to multiply the denominators: For 2/5 + 1/2 multiply 5 by 2. Now you have a denominator of 10. However, now you have to change the top numbers too. Since you multiplied the 5 in 2/5 by 2, you also multiply the 2 by 2, to get 4. So the first number is now 4/10. Since you multiplied the second number times 5, you also multiply its top number by 5, to get a final fraction of 5/10. Now you can add 5 and 4 together to get a final sum of 9/10.

- Sometimes you'll be asked to reduce a fraction to its simplest form. This means getting it to where the only common factor of the numerator and denominator is 1. Think of it this way: Numerators and denominators are brothers that must be treated the same. If you do something to one, you must do it to the other, or it's just not fair. For instance, if you divide your numerator by 2, then you should also divide the denominator by the same. Let's take an example: The fraction 2/10 . This is not reduced to its simplest terms because there is a number that will divide evenly into both: the number 2. We want to make it so that the only number that will divide evenly into both is 1. What can we divide into 2 to get 1? The number 2, of course! Now to be "fair," we have to do the same thing to the denominator: Divide 2 into 10 and you get 5. So our new, reduced fraction is 1/5.

- In some ways, multiplying fractions is the easiest of all: Just multiply the two top numbers and then multiply the two bottom numbers. For instance, with this problem:
2/5 X 2/3 you multiply 2 by 2 and get a top number of 4; then multiply 5 by 3 and get a bottom number of 15. Your answer is 4/15.

- Dividing fractions is more involved, but still not too hard. You once again multiply, but only AFTER you have turned the second fraction upside-down. To divide ⅞ by ½, turn the ½ into 2/1, then multiply the top numbers and multiply the bottom numbers: ⅞ X 2/1 gives us 14 on top and 8 on the bottom.

## Converting Fractions to Decimals

There are a couple of ways to become good at converting fractions to decimals. One -- the one that will make you the fastest in basic math skills -- is to learn some basic fraction facts. It's a good idea, if you're good at memory, to memorize the following:

1/100 is "one hundredth," expressed as a decimal, it's .01.

1/50 is "two hundredths," expressed as a decimal, it's .02.

1/25 is "one twenty-fifths" or "four hundredths," expressed as a decimal, it's .04.

1/20 is "one twentieth" or ""five hundredths," expressed as a decimal, it's .05.

1/10 is "one tenth," expressed as a decimal, it's .1.

1/8 is "one eighth," or "one hundred twenty-five thousandths," expressed as a decimal, it's .125.

1/5 is "one fifth," or "two tenths," expressed as a decimal, it's .2.

1/4 is "one fourth" or "twenty-five hundredths," expressed as a decimal, it's .25.

1/3 is "one third" or "thirty-three hundredths," expressed as a decimal, it's .33.

1/2 is "one half" or "five tenths," expressed as a decimal, it's .5.

3/4 is "three fourths," or "seventy-five hundredths," expressed as a decimal, it's .75.

Of course, if you're no good at memorization, another good technique for converting a fraction to a decimal is to manipulate it so that the fraction's denominator is 10, 10, 1000, or some other power of 10. Here's an example: We'll start with ¾. What is the first number in the 4 "times table" that you can multiply and get a multiple of 10? Can you multiply 4 by something to get 10? No. Can you multiply it by something to get 100? Yes! 4 X 25 is 100. So let's take that 25 and multiply it by the numerator in our fraction ¾. The numerator is 3, and 3 X 25 is 75. We'll move the decimal in 75 all the way to the left, and we find that ¾ is .75.

We'll do another one: 1/5. Again, we want to find a power of 10 that 5 goes into evenly. Will 5 go into 10? Yes! It goes 2 times. So we'll take that 2 and multiply it by our numerator, 1, and we get 2. We move the decimal in 2 all the way to the left and find that 1/5 is equal to .2.

## Converting Fractions to Percent

Here is a quick method to convert fraction to percent and a strategy for answering on a multiple choice test that will save you valuable exam time.

First, remember that a fraction is a division problem: you're dividing the bottom number into the top.

Taking an example, convert 2/3 into percent.

The first method is to multiple the numerator by 100 and divide. So,

(2 X 100) / 2 = 100/3 = 66.66

Add a % sign and you have the answer, 66.66%

If you're doing these conversions on a multiple-choice test, here's an idea that might be even easier and faster. Let's say you have a fraction of 1/8 and you're asked to convert to percent.

Since we know that "percent" means hundredths, ask yourself what number we can multiply 8 by to get 100. Since there is no number, ask what number gets us close to 100.

That number is 12: 8 X 12 = 96. So it gets us a little less than 100. Now, whatever you do to the denominator, you have to do to the numerator. Let's multiply 1 X 12 and we get 12. However, since 96 is a little less than 100, we know that our answer will be a little MORE than 12%.

Look at the choices and eliminate the obvious wrong choices. So if your possible answers on the multiple-choice test are these:

a) 8.5%  b) 19%  c) 12.5%  d) 25%

then we know the answer is c) 12.5%, because it's a little MORE than the 12 we got in our math problem above.

Here all the choices except choice C 12.5% can be eliminated.

You don't have to know the exact correct answer, just enough to estimate, then eliminate the obviously wrong answers.

This was an easy example to demonstrate the strategy, but don't be fooled! You probably won't get such an easy question on your exam. By estimating your answer quickly, then eliminating obviously incorrect choices immediately, you save precious exam time.

## Decimal Tips, Tricks and Short-cuts

## Converting Decimals to Fractions

Converting decimals to fractions is easy if you say it the right way! If you say "point one" or "point 25," you'll have trouble.

But if you say, "one tenth" and "twenty-five hundredths," then you have already solved it! That's because, if you know your fractions, you know that "one tenth" looks like this: 1/10. And "twenty-five hundredths" looks like this: 25/100.

Even if you have digits before the decimal, such as 3.4, learning how to say the word will help you with the conversion into a fraction. It's not "three point four," it's "three and four tenths." Knowing this, you know that the fraction which looks like "three and four tenths" is 3 4/10.

The conversion is not complete until you reduce the fraction to its lowest terms: It's not 25/100, but 1/4.

## Converting Decimals to Percent

Changing a decimal to a percent is easy if you remember one thing: multiply by 100.

For example, if you start with .45, simply multiply it by 100 for 45. Then add the % sign to the end - 45%.

Think of it this way: take out the decimal point, add a percent sign on the opposite side. In other words, the decimal on the left is replaced by the % on the right.

It doesn't work quite that easily if the decimal is in the middle of the number. For example, 3.7. Here, take out the decimal in the middle and replace it with a 0 % at the end. So 3.7 converted to decimal is 370%.

## Percent Tips, Tricks and Shortcuts

Percent problems are not nearly as scary as they appear, if you remember this neat trick:

Draw a cross as in:

|  Portion  |  Percent  |
|-----------|-----------|
|  Whole    |  100      |

In the upper left, write PORTION. In the bottom left, write WHOLE. In the top right, write PERCENT and in the bottom right, write 100. Whatever your problem is, you will leave blank the unknown, and fill in the other four parts. For example, let's suppose your problem is: Find 10% of 50. Since we know the 10% part, we put 10 in the percent corner. Since the whole number in our problem is 50, we put that in the corner marked whole. You always put 100 underneath the percent, so we leave it as is, which leaves only the top left corner blank. This is where we'll put our answer. Now simply multiply the two corner numbers that are NOT 100. Here, it's 10 X 50. That gives us 500. Now divide this by the remaining corner, or 100, to get a final answer of 5. 5 is the number that goes in the upper-left corner, and is your final solution.

Another hint to remember: Percents are the same thing as hundredths in decimals. So .45 is the same as 45 hundredths or 45 percent.

### Converting Percents to Decimals

Percent are a type of decimal, so it should be no surprise that converting between the two is actually fairly simple. Here are a few tricks and shortcuts to keep in mind:

- Remember that percent literally means "per 100" or "for every 100." So when you speak of 30% you're saying 30 for every 100 or the fraction 30/100. In basic math, you learned that fractions that have 10 or 100 as the denominator can easily be turned to a decimal. 30/100 is thirty hundredths, or expressed as a decimal, .30.
- Another way to look at it: To convert a percent to a decimal, simply divide the number by 100. So for instance, if the percent is 47%, divide 47 by 100. The result will be .47. Get rid of the % mark and you're done.
- Remember that the easiest way of dividing by 100 is by moving your decimal two spots to the left.

### Converting Percent to Fractions

Converting Percent to Fractions is easy. After all, a percent is just a type of fraction;

it tells you what part of 100 that you're talking about. Here are some simple ideas for making the conversion from a percent to a fraction:

- If the percent is a whole number -- say 34% -- then simply write a fraction with 100 as the denominator (the bottom number). Then put the percentage itself on top. So 34% becomes 34/100.
- Now reduce as you would reduce any percent. Here, by dividing 2 into 34 and 2 into 100, you get 17/50.
- If your percent is not a whole number -- say 3.4% --then convert it to a decimal expressed as hundredths. 3.4 is the same as 3.40 (or 3 and forty hundredths). Now ask yourself how you would express "three and forty hundredths" as a fraction. It would, of course, be 3 40/100. Reduce this and it becomes 3 2/5.

## How to Answer Basic Math Multiple Choice

Math is the one section where you need to make sure that you understand the processes before you ever tackle it. That's because the time allowed on the math portion is typically so short that there's not much room for error. You have to be fast and accurate. It's imperative that before the test day arrives, you've learned all the main formulas that will be used, and then to create your own problems (and solve them).

On the actual test day, use the "Plug-Check-Check" strategy. Here's how it goes.

Read the problem, but not the answers. You'll want to work the problem first and come up with your own answers. If you did the work right, you should find your answer among the choices given.

If you need help with the problem, plug actual numbers into the variables given. You'll find it easier to work with numbers than it is to work with letters. For instance, if the question asks, "If Y - 4 is 2 more than Z, then Y + 5 is how much more than Z?" Try selecting a value for Y. Let's take 6. Your question now becomes, "If 6 - 4 is 2 more than Z, then 6 plus 5 is how much more than Z?" Now your answer should be easier to work with.

Check the answer choices to see if your answer matches one of those. If so, select it.

If no answer matches the one you got, re-check your math, but this time, use a different method. In math, it's common for there to be more than one way to solve a problem. As a simple example, if you multiplied 12 X 13 and did not get an answer that matches one of the answer choices, you might try adding 13 together 12 different times and see if you get a good answer.

## Math Multiple Choice Strategy

The two strategies for working with basic math multiple choice are Estimation and Elimination.

**Math Strategy 1 - Estimation.**

Just like it sounds, try to estimate an approximate answer first. Then look at the choices.

**Math Strategy 2 - Elimination.**

For every question, no matter what type, eliminating obviously incorrect answers narrows the possible choices. Elimination is probably the most powerful strategy for answering multiple choice.

Here are a few basic math examples.

**Solve 2/3 + 5/12**

    a. 9/17

    b. 3/11

    c. 7/12

    d. 1 1/12

First estimate the answer. 2/3 is more than half and 5/12 is about half, so the answer is going to be very close to 1.

Next, Eliminate. Choice A is about 1/2 and can be eliminated, choice B is very small, less than 1/2 and can be eliminated. Choice C is close to 1/2 and can be eliminated. Leaving only choice D, which is just over 1.

Work through the solution, a common denominator is needed, a number which both 3 and 12 will divide into.
2/3 = 8/12. So, 8+5/12 = 13/12 = 1 1/12

Choice D is correct.

**Solve 4/5 – 2/3**

    a. 2/2

    b. 2/13

    c. 1

    d. 2/15

You can eliminate choice A, because it is 1 and since both numbers are close to one, the difference is going to be very small. You can eliminate choice C for the same reason.

Next, look at the denominators. Since 5 and 3 don't go into 13, you can eliminate choice B as well.

That leaves choice D.

Checking the answer, the common denominator will be 15. So 12-10/15 = 2/15. Choice D is correct.

**Fractions shortcut - Cancelling out.**

In any operation with fractions, if the numerator of one fraction has a common multiple with the denominator of the other, you can cancel out. This saves time, and simplifies the problem quickly, making it easier to manage.

**Solve 2/15 ÷ 4/5**

    a. 6/65

    b. 6/75

    c. 5/12

    d. 1/6

To divide fractions, we multiply the first fraction with the inverse of the second fraction. Therefore we have
2/15 x 5/4. The numerator of the first fraction, 2, shares a multiple with the denominator of the second fraction, 4, which is 2. These cancel out, which gives, 1/3 x 1/2 = 1/6

Cancelling out solved the questions very quickly, but we can still use multiple choice strategies to answer.

Choice B can be eliminated because 75 is too large a denominator. Choice C can be eliminated because 5 and 15 don't go into 12.

Choice D is correct.

**Decimal Multiple Choice Strategy and Shortcuts.**

Multiplying decimals gives a very quick way to estimate and eliminate choices. Anytime that you multiply decimals, it is going to give an answer with the same number of decimal places as the combined operands.

So for example,

2.38 X 1.2 will produce a number with three places of decimal, which is 2.856.

Here are a few examples with step-by-step explanation:

**Solve 2.06 x 1.2**

    a. 24.82

    b. 2.482

    c. 24.72

    d. 2.472

This is a simple question, but even before you start calculating, you can eliminate several choices. When multiplying decimals, there will always be as many numbers behind the decimal place in the answer as the sum of the ones in the initial problem, so choices A and C can be eliminated.

The correct answer is D: 2.06 x 1.2 = 2.472

**Solve 20.0 ÷ 2.5**

    a. 12.05

    b. 9.25

    c. 8.3

    d. 8

First estimate the answer to be around 10, and eliminate choice A. And since it'd also be an even number, you can eliminate choices B and C, leaving only choice D.

The correct Answer is D: 20.0 ÷ 2.5 = 8

## How to Solve Word Problems

Most students find math word problems difficult. Solving word problems is much easier if you have a systematic approach which we outline below.

Here is the biggest tip for studying word problems.

**Practice regularly and systematically.** Sounds simple and easy right? Yes it is, and yes it really does work.

Word problems are a way of thinking and require you to translate a real world problem into mathematical terms.

Some math instructors go so far as to say that learning how to think mathematically is the main reason for teaching word problems.

So what do we mean by practice regularly and systematically? Studying word problems and math in general requires a logical and mathematical frame of mind. The only way that you can get this is by practicing regularly, which means everyday.

It is critical that you practice word problems everyday for the 5 days before the exam as a bare minimum.

If you practice and miss a day, you have lost the mathematical frame of mind and the benefit of your previous practice is pretty much gone. Anyone who has done math will agree – you have to practice everyday.

**Everything is important.** The other critical point about word problems is that all the information given in the problem has some purpose. There is no unnecessary information! Word problems are typically around 50 words in 1 to 3 sentences. If the sometimes complicated relationships are to be explained in that short an explanation, every word has to count. Make sure that you use every piece of information.

**Here are 9 simple steps to help you resolve word problems.**

**Step 1** – Read through the problem at least three times. The first reading should be a quick scan, and the next two readings should be done slowly to find answers to these questions:

What does the problem ask? (Usually located towards the end of the problem)

What does the problem imply? (This is usually a point you were asked to remember).

Mark all information, and underline all important words or phrases.

**Step 2** – Try to make a pictorial representation of the problem such as a circle and an arrow to show travel. This makes the problem a bit more real and sensible to you.

A favorite word problem is something like, 1 train leaves Station A travelling at 100 km/hr and another leaves Station B travelling at 60 km/hr. ...

Draw a line, the two stations, and the two trains at either end. This will clarify the problem.

**Step 3** – Use the information you have to make a table with a blank portion to show information you do not know.

**Step 4** – Assign a single letter to represent each unknown data in your table. You can write down the unknown that each letter represents so that you do not make the error of assigning answers to the wrong unknown, because a word problem may have multiple unknowns and you will need to create equations for each unknown.

**Step 5** – Translate the English terms in the word problem into a mathematical algebraic equation. Remember that the main problem with word problems is that they are not expressed in regular math equations. You ability to correctly identify the variables and translate the word problem into an equation determines your ability to solve the problem.

**Step 6** – Check the equation to see if it looks like regular equations that you are used to seeing, and if it looks sensible. Does the equation appear to represent the information in the question? Take note that you may need to rewrite some formulas needed to solve the word problem equation. For example, word distance problems may require rewriting the distance formula, Distance = Time x Rate. If the word problem requires a solution for time, use Distance/Rate and Distance/Time to solve for Rate. If you understand the distance word problem you should be able to identify the variable you need to solve for.

**Step 7** – Use algebra rules to solve the derived equation. Take note that the laws of equation demands that what is done on this side of the equation has to also be done on the other side. You have to solve the equation so that the unknown ends alone on one side. Where there are multiple unknowns you will need to use elimination or substitution methods to resolve all the equations.

**Step 8** – Check your final answers to see if they make sense with the information given in the problem. For example if the word problem involves a discount, the final price should be less or if a product was taxed then the final answer has to cost more.

**Step 9** – Cross check your answers by placing the answer or answers in the first equation to replace the unknown or unknowns. If your answer is correct then both sides of the equation must equate or equal. If your answer is not correct then you may have derived a wrong equation or solved the equation wrongly. Repeat the necessary steps to correct.

## Types of Word Problems

Word problems can be classified into 12 types. Below are examples of each type with a complete solution. Some types of word problems can be solved quickly using multiple choice strategies and some cannot. Always look for ways to estimate the answer and then eliminate choices.

### 1. Age

A girl is 10 years older than her brother. By next year, she will be twice the age of her brother. What are their ages now?

    a. 25, 15
    b. 19, 9
    c. 21, 11
    d. 29, 19

**Solution:** B

We will assume that the girl's age is "a" and her brother's is "b." This means that based on the information in the first sentence, a = 10 + b

Next year, she will be twice her brother's age, which gives
a + 1 = 2(b + 1)

We need to solve for one unknown factor and then use the answer to solve for the other. To do this we substitute the value of "a" from the first equation into the second equation. This gives

10 + b + 1 = 2b + 2
11 + b = 2b + 2
11 − 2 = 2b − b
b = 9

9 = b this means that her brother is 9 years old.
Solving for the girl's age in the first equation gives

a = 10 + 9
a = 19 the girl is aged 19. So, the girl is aged 19 and the boy is 9

## 2. Distance or Speed

Two boats travel down a river towards the same destination, starting at the same time. One boat is traveling at 52 km/hr, and the other boat at 43 km/hr. How far apart will they be after 40 minutes?

   a. 46.67 km
   b. 19.23 km
   c. 6 km
   d. 14.39 km

**Solution:** C

After 40 minutes, the first boat will have traveled = 52 km/hr x 40 minutes/60 minutes = 34.66 km
After 40 minutes, the second boat will have traveled = 43 km/hr x 40/60 minutes = 28.66 km
Difference between the two boats will be 34.66 km − 28.66 km = 6 km.

**Multiple Choice Strategy**

First estimate the answer. The first boat is travelling 9 km. faster than the second, for 40 minutes, which is 2/3 of an hour. 2/3 of 9 = 6, as a rough guess of the distance apart.

Choices A, B and D can be eliminated right away.

## 3. Ratio

A recipe state that 700 grams of flour must be mixed in 100 ml of water, and 0.90 grams of salt added. A cook however has just 325 grams of flour. How much water and salt should be used?

    a. 0.41 grams and 46.4 ml

    b. 0.45 grams and 49.3 ml

    c. 0.39 grams and 39.8 ml

    d. 0.25 grams and 40.1 ml

**Solution:** A

The Cookbook states 700 grams of flour, but the cook only has 325. The first step is to determine the percentage of flour he has 325/700 x 100 = 46.4%
That means that 46.4% of all other items must also be used.
46.4% of 100 = 46.4 ml of water
46.4% of 0.90 = 0.41 grams of salt.

**Multiple Choice Strategy**

The recipe calls for 700 grams of flour but the cook only has 325, which is just less than half, the quantity of water and salt are going to be approximately half.

Choices C and D can be eliminated right away. Choice B is very close so be careful. Looking closely at choice B, it is exactly half, and since 325 is slightly less than half of 700, it can't be correct.

Choice A is correct.

## 4. Percent

An agent received $6,685 as his commission for selling a property. If his commission was 13% of the selling price, how much was the property?

    a. $68,825

    b. $121,850

    c. $49,025

    d. $51,423

**Solution:** D

Let's assume that the property price is x
That means from the information given, 13% of x = 6,685
Solve for x,
x = 6685 x 100/13 = $51,423

**Multiple Choice Strategy**

The commission, 13%, is just over 10%, which is easier to work with. Round up $6685 to $6700, and multiple by 10 for an approximate answer. 10 X 6700 = $67,000. You can do this in your head. Choice B is much too big and can be eliminated. Choice C is too small and can be eliminated. Choices A and D are left and good possibilities.

Do the calculations to make the final choice.

## 5. Sales & Profit

A store owner buys merchandise for $21,045. He transports them for $3,905 and pays his staff $1,450 to stock the merchandise on his shelves. If he does not incur further costs, how much does he need to sell the items to make $5,000 profit?

   a. $32,500
   b. $29,350
   c. $32,400
   d. $31,400

**Solution:** D

Total cost of the items is $21,045 + $3,905 + $1,450 = $26,400
Total cost is now $26,400 + $5000 profit = $31,400

**Multiple Choice Strategy**

Round off and add the numbers up in your head quickly.
21,000 + 4,000 + 1500 = 26500. Add in 5000 profit for a total of 31500.

Choice B is too small and can be eliminated. Choice C and Choice A are too large and can be eliminated.

## 6. Tax/Income

A woman earns $42,000 per month and pays 5% tax on her monthly income. If the Government increases her monthly taxes by $1,500, what is her income after tax?

   a. $38,400
   b. $36,050
   c. $40,500
   d. $39, 500

**Solution:** A

Initial tax on income was 5/100 x 42,000 = $2,100
$1,500 was added to the tax to give $2,100 + 1,500 = $3,600
Income after tax left is $42,000 - $3,600 = $38,400

## 7. Interest

A man invests $3000 in a 2-year term deposit that pays 3% interest per year. How much will he have at the end of the 2-year term?

    a. $5,200
    b. $3,020
    c. $3,182.7
    d. $3,000

**Solution:** C

This is a compound interest problem. The funds are invested for 2 years and interest is paid yearly, so in the second year, he will earn interest on the interest paid in the first year.

3% interest in the first year = 3/100 x 3,000 = $90
At end of first year, total amount = 3,000 + 90 = $3,090
Second year = 3/100 x 3,090 = 92.7.
At end of second year, total amount = $3090 + $92.7 = $3,182.7

## 8. Averaging

The average weight of 10 books is 54 grams. 2 more books were added and the average weight became 55.4. If one of the 2 new books added weighed 62.8 g, what is the weight of the other?

    a. 44.7 g
    b. 67.4 g
    c. 62 g
    d. 52 g

**Solution:** C

Total weight of 10 books with average 54 grams will be = 10 × 54 = 540 g
Total weight of 12 books with average 55.4 will be = 55.4 × 12 = 664.8 g
So total weight of the remaining 2 will be= 664.8 – 540 = 124.8 g
If one weighs 62.8, the weight of the other will be= 124.8 g – 62.8 g = 62 g

**Multiple Choice Strategy**

Averaging problems can be estimated by looking at which direction the average goes. If additional items are added and the average goes up, the new items much be greater than the average. If the average goes down after new items are added, the new items must be less than the average.

Here, the average is 54 grams and 2 books are added which increases the average to

55.4, so the new books must weight more than 54 grams.

Choices A and D can be eliminated right away.

## 9. Probability

A bag contains 15 marbles of various colors. If 3 marbles are white, 5 are red and the rest are black, what is the probability of randomly picking out a black marble from the bag?

   a. 7/15
   b. 3/15
   c. 1/5
   d. 4/15

**Solution:** A

Total marbles = 15
Number of black marbles = 15 – (3 + 5) = 7
Probability of picking out a black marble = 7/15

## 10. Two Variables

A company paid a total of $2850 to book for 6 single rooms and 4 double rooms in a hotel for one night. Another company paid $3185 to book for 13 single rooms for one night in the same hotel. What is the cost for single and double rooms in that hotel?

   a. single= $250 and double = $345
   b. single= $254 and double = $350
   c. single = $245 and double = $305
   d. single = $245 and double = $345

**Solution:** D

We can determine the price of single rooms from the information given of the second company. 13 single rooms = 3185.
One single room = 3185 / 13 = 245
The first company paid for 6 single rooms at $245. 245 x 6 = $1470
Total amount paid for 4 double rooms by first company = $2850 - $1470 = $1380
Cost per double room = 1380 / 4 = $345

## 11. Geometry

The length of a rectangle is 5 in. more than its width. The perimeter of the rectangle is 26 in. What is the width and length of the rectangle?

    a. width = 6 inches, Length = 9 inches
    b. width = 4 inches, Length = 9 inches
    c. width =4 inches, Length = 5 inches
    d. width = 6 inches, Length = 11 inches

**Solution:** B

Formula for perimeter of a rectangle is 2(L + W)
p=26, so 2(L+W) = p
The length is 5 inches more than the width, so
2(w+5) + 2w = 26
2w + 10 + 2w = 26
2w + 2w = 26 - 10
4w = 166

W = 16/4 = 4 inches

L is 5 inches more than w, so L = 5 + 4 = 9 inches.


## 12. Totals and fractions

A basket contains 125 oranges, mangos and apples. If 3/5 of the fruits in the basket are mangos and only 2/5 of the mangos are ripe, how many ripe mangos are there in the basket?

    a. 30
    b. 68
    c. 55
    d. 47

**Solution:** A
Number of mangos in the basket is 3/5 x 125 = 75
Number of ripe mangos = 2/5 x 75 = 30

# Exponents: Tips, Shortcuts & Tricks

Exponents seem like advanced math to most—like some mysterious code with a complicated meaning. In fact, though, an exponent is just short hand for saying that you're multiplying a number by itself two or more times. For instance, instead of saying that you're multiplying 5 x 5 x 5, you can show that you're multiplying 5 by itself 3 times if you just write $5^3$. We usually say this as "five to the third power" or "five to the power of three." In this example, the raised 3 is an "exponent," while the 5 is the "base." You can even use exponents with fractions. For instance, $½^3$ means you're multiplying ½ x ½ x ½. (The answer is 1/8). Some other helpful hints for working with exponents:

Here's how to do basic multiplication of exponents. If you have the same number with a different exponent (For instance $5^3$ X $5^2$) just add the exponents and multiply the bases as usual. The answer, then, is $5^5$.

This doesn't work, though, if the bases are different. For instance, in $5^3$ X $3^2$ we simply have to do the math the long way to figure out the final solution: 5 x 5 x 5, multiplying by the result for 3 X 2. (The answer is 750).

Looking at it from the opposite side, to divide two exponents with the same base (or bottom number), subtract the smaller exponent from the larger one. If we were dividing the problem above, we would subtract the 2 from the 3 to get 1. 5 to the power of 1 is simply 5.

One time when thinking of exponents as merely multiplication doesn't work is when the raised number is zero. Any number raised to the "zeroth" power is 1 (Not, as we tend to think, zero).

| Number (x) | $x^2$ | $x^3$ |
|---|---|---|
| 1 | 1 | 1 |
| 2 | 4 | 8 |
| 3 | 9 | 27 |
| 4 | 16 | 64 |
| 5 | 25 | 125 |
| 6 | 36 | 216 |
| 7 | 49 | 343 |
| 8 | 64 | 512 |
| 9 | 81 | 729 |
| 10 | 100 | 1000 |

## Mean, Median and Mode

Mean, mode and median are basic statistical tools used to calculate different types of averages.

### Mean

Mean is the most common form of average used. To calculate mean, you simple add up all the values of data given and divide by the number data provided.

**Example**

Find the mean of 8, 5, 7, 10, 15, 21
Sum of values = 8 + 5 + 7 + 10 + 15 + 21 = 66
Number of data = 6
Mean = 66/6 = 11

### Median

Median refers to the middle value among a set or series of values after they have been arranged in numerical order. Median thus means the middle of the set of values. When two numbers fall in the middle, you simple add the value of the two numbers and divide by 2 to get the middle of the two numbers.

**Example**

Arrange these numbers in ascending order and then find the median

First arrange in ascending order 8, 5, 7, 10, 15, 21
= 5, 7, 8, 10, 15, 21

There are 6 numbers on the series and two fall in the middle = 8 and 10
The median = 8 + 10/2
= 18/2 =9

### Mode

Mode refers to the most occurring number or value among a set of values. Note that it is possible not to have a most occurring number and then the answer becomes 'No Mode'

**Example**

8, 5, 7, 10, 15, 21, 5, 7, 2, 5

Mode refers to the most occurring number
8, 10, 15, 2 and 21 occur once

5 occurs 3 times
7 occurs 2 times

The most occurring number is 5, which occurs three times.

## Order Of Operation

Some math calculations contain more than one set of operations. For example, a problem like 3 + (35 - 21) x 2 requires addition, subtraction and multiplication operations. The problem arises from the confusion of which of the operations to perform first. Starting with the wrong operation will give you the wrong answer. To solve this dilemma and to avoid confusion, the Order of Operation rules were set.

Order of operation is a set of mathematical rules designed to be used for calculations that require more than one arithmetic operation. For example, calculation problems that require two or more out of addition, subtraction, multiplication and division, would require that you follow the order of operation to solve.

The order of operation rules are simple as explained below.

> **Rule 1:** Start with calculations that are inside brackets or parentheses.
> **Rule 2:** Then, solve all multiplications and divisions, from left to right.
> **Rule 3:** Finally, solve all additions and subtractions, from left to right.

**Example 1**

Solve 16 + 5 x 8

Based on the rules above, we would have to start with the multiplication part of the question.
That will give: 16 + 40 = 56

Take note that if the rule was not followed and addition was done first, the answer gotten would be different and wrong.

16 + 5 x 8
21 x 8 = 168 (wrong answer)

**Example 2**

3 +(35 - 21) x 2

Based on the rules of the order of operation, we have to solve the problem in the bracket or parenthesis first. Then we do the multiplication, before doing the addition.

3 + (35 - 21) x 2
3 + (14) x 2
3 + 28
=31

## Scientific Notation

Scientific notation is a very simple and effective way of representing very large numbers in simpler forms. For example, instead of writing out 149,600,000,000 meters, which is the estimated distance from the sun, astronomers could easily write it out as $1.496 \times 10^{11}$ meters.

Scientific notation expresses numbers in their powers of ten. It can be used to even express simple numbers.

For example, using scientific notation, $10 = 10^1$ The exponent "1" tells the number of times to multiply by 10 to get the original number.
$100 = 10^2$
$1000 = 10^3$
$10^0 = 1$

When the exponent is negative, it tells us how many times we need to divide by ten to get the original number.

For example, $0.025 = 2.5 \times 10$

The accepted format of scientific notation or writing numbers on their powers of 10 is a $\times 10^n$
Where a must be between 1 and 10 and n must be an integer

**How to convert to scientific notation**

To convert a number to scientific notation, you would need to place a decimal after the first number that is not a zero or after the first number that ranges between 1 and 9.

After placing the decimal, you need to count the number of places that the decimal had to move to get the exponent of 10. If the decimal moves to the left, then the exponent to multiply 10 will be in the positive. If the decimal moves from right to left, we will then have a negative power of 10.

For example, to convert 29010, we need to place a decimal after 2, since 2 is the first non zero number. We would then have 2.91

If we were to convert 0.0167, we need to place the decimal after 1, since the first two numbers before 1 were zeros and do not fall between 1 and 9. We would thus have 1.67

To complete the conversion of 29010 to scientific notation, we would get $2.91 \times 10^4$

The 10 is raised to the power of 4, because there are 4 places counting from the right to left where the decimal had to move. This scientific notation is in the positive because the decimal moved to the left.

$0.0167 = 1.67 \times 10^{-2}$

In this example, the decimal place moved from left to right by 2 spaces thus the 10 is raised to the power of 2. It is in the negative, because the decimal moved towards the right.

**How to convert from scientific notation**

You may also need to convert numbers that are already represented in scientific notation or in their power of ten to regular numbers. It is quite easy.

First it is important to remember these two laws.

If the power is in the positive, shift decimal to the right
If the power is in the negative, shift decimal point to the left

**Example**

Convert $3.201 \times 10^3$

This scientific notation is in the positive so we just need to shift the decimal to the right by 2 spaces, which is the power of the 10. We thus have: $3.201 \times 10^3 = 3201$

**Another example**

Convert

$1.03 \times 10^{-4}$

The scientific notation here is negative and so we need to shift decimal to the left. Thus $1.03 \times 10^{-2} = 0.000103$ The decimal was shifted 4 spaces to the left.

## Ratios

In mathematics, a ratio is a relationship between two numbers of the same kind (e.g., objects, persons, students, spoonfuls, units of whatever identical dimension), usually expressed as "a to b" or a:b, sometimes expressed arithmetically as a dimensionless quotient of the two which explicitly indicates how many times the first number contains the second (not necessarily an integer).In layman's terms a ratio represents, for every amount of one thing, how much there is of another thing. For example, suppose I have 10 pairs of socks for every pair of shoes then the ratio of shoes:socks would be 1:10 and the ratio of socks:shoes would be 10:1.

**Notation and terminology**

The ratio of numbers A and B can be expressed as: the ratio of A to B
A is to B
A:B

A rational number which is the quotient of A divided by B
The numbers A and B are sometimes called terms with A being the antecedent and B being the consequent.

The proportion expressing the equality of the ratios A:B and C:D is written A:B=C:D or A:B::C:D. This latter form, when spoken or written in the English language, is often expressed as
A is to B as C is to D.

Again, A, B, C, D are called the terms of the proportion. A and D are called the extremes, and B and C are called the means. The equality of three or more proportions is called a continued proportion.[5]
Ratios are sometimes used with three or more terms. The dimensions of a two by four that is ten inches long are 2:4:10.

**Examples**

The quantities being compared in a ratio might be physical quantities such as speed or length, or numbers of objects, or amounts of particular substances. A common example of the last case is the weight ratio of water to cement used in concrete, which is commonly stated as 1:4. This means that the weight of cement used is four times the weight of water used. It does not say anything about the total amounts of cement and water used, nor the amount of concrete being made. Equivalently it could be said that the ratio of cement to water is 4:1, that there is 4 times as much cement as water, or that there is a quarter (1/4) as much water as cement.

Older televisions have a 4:3 "aspect ratio," which means that the width is 4/3 of the height; modern widescreen TVs have a 16:9 aspect ratio.

## Fractional

If there are 2 oranges and 3 apples, the ratio of oranges to apples is 2:3, and the ratio of oranges to the total number of pieces of fruit is 2:5. These ratios can also be expressed in fraction form: there are 2/3 as many oranges as apples, and 2/5 of the pieces of fruit are oranges. If orange juice concentrate is to be diluted with water in the ratio 1:4, then one part of concentrate is mixed with four parts of water, giving five parts total; the amount of orange juice concentrate is 1/4 the amount of water, while the amount of orange juice concentrate is 1/5 of the total liquid. In both ratios and fractions, it is important to be clear what is being compared to what, and beginners often make mistakes for this reason.
**Number of terms**

In general, when comparing the quantities of a two-quantity ratio, this can be expressed as a fraction derived from the ratio. For example, in a ratio of 2:3, the amount/size/volume/number of the first quantity will be that of the second quantity. This pattern also works with ratios with more than two terms. However, a ratio with more than two terms cannot be completely converted into a single fraction; a single fraction represents only one part of the ratio since a fraction can only compare two numbers. If the ratio deals with objects or amounts of objects, this is often expressed as "for every two parts of the first quantity there are three parts of the second quantity."

## Percent and ratio

Multiplying a ratio by a number, the ratio remains valid. For example, the ratio of 6:3 is the same as 12:6. It is usual either to reduce terms to the lowest common denominator, or to express them in parts per hundred (percent).

If a mixture contains substances A, B, C & D in the ratio 5:9:4:2 then there are 5 parts of A for every 9 parts of B, 4 parts of C and 2 parts of D. As 5+9+4+2=20, the total mixture contains 5/20 of A (5 parts out of 20), 9/20 of B, 4/20 of C, and 2/20 of D. If we divide all numbers by the total and multiply by 100, this is converted to percentages: 25% A, 45% B, 20% C, and 10% D (equivalent to writing the ratio as 25:45:20:10).

## Proportion

If the two or more ratio quantities encompass all the quantities in a particular situation, for example two apples and three oranges in a fruit basket containing no other types of fruit, it could be said that "the whole" contains five parts, made up of two parts apples and three parts oranges. Here, or 40% of the whole are apples or 60% of the whole are oranges. This comparison of a specific quantity to "the whole" is sometimes called a proportion. Proportions are sometimes expressed as percentages as demonstrated above.

## Reduction

Note that ratios can be reduced (as fractions are) by dividing each quantity by the common factors of all the quantities. This is often called "cancelling." As for fractions, the simplest form is considered to be that in which the numbers in the ratio are the smallest possible integers.

Thus, the ratio 40:60 may be considered equivalent in meaning to the ratio 2:3 within contexts concerned only with relative quantities.

Mathematically, we write: "40:60" = "2:3" (dividing both quantities by 20).
Grammatically, we would say, "40 to 60 equals 2 to 3."
An alternative representation is: "40:60::2:3"
Grammatically, we would say, "40 is to 60 as 2 is to 3."
A ratio that has integers for both quantities and that cannot be reduced any further (using integers) is said to be in simplest form or lowest terms.
Sometimes it is useful to write a ratio in the form 1:n or n:1 to enable comparisons of different ratios.

For example, the ratio 4:5 can be written as 1:1.25 (dividing both sides by 4). Alternatively, 4:5 can be written as 0.8:1 (dividing both sides by 5). Where the context makes the meaning clear, a ratio in this form is sometimes written without the 1 and the colon, though, mathematically, this makes it a factor or multiplier.

## Perimeter Area and Volume

### Definitions

**Perimeter** - the linear distance around a figure

**Area** - the number of square units to completely cover a 2-D face

**Surface Area** - the combined areas of all faces of a 3-D solid

**Volume** - The number of cube units to completely fill a 3-D solid

### Perimeter and Area (2-dimentional shapes)

Perimeter of a shape determines the length around that shape, while the area includes the space inside the shape.

### Example Problems

**Determine the Perimeter of a 2-D Shape**
To determine the perimeter of any figure, simply add the lengths of every side. Be sure to write you final answer with linear units.

Rectangles have opposite sides that are congruent (exactly the same), so an alternate method is to double the sum of the length and width.

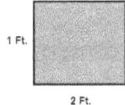

Identify the opposite sides are congruent.

Add all sides.

P = 2 + 1 + 2 + 1 = 6 ft

### Determine the Area of a 2-D Shape

Specific equations exist to determine the areas of basic 2-D figures. When multiple figures are present, select the equation appropriate to your figure, and then substitute values and solve. Be sure that your final answer has square units.

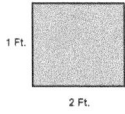

$Area_{Rectangle}$ = Length * Width
$Area_{Rectangle}$ = (2 ft)·(1 ft)
$Area_{Rectangle}$ = 2 ft²

### Common 2-D figures and formula for Area and Perimeter

**Rectangle:**

$P = 2a + 2b$
$A = ab$

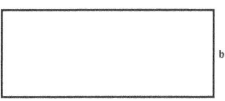

**Square**

$P = 4a$
$A = a^2$

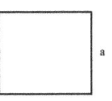

**Parallelogram**

$P = 2a + 2b$
$A = ah_a = bh_b$

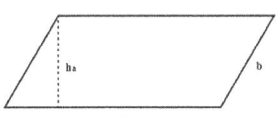

### Rhombus

$P = 4a$

$A = ah = \dfrac{d_1 d_2}{2}$

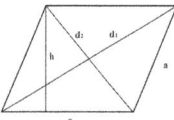

### Triangle

$P = a + b + c$

$A = \dfrac{ah_a}{2} = \dfrac{bh_b}{2} = \dfrac{ch_c}{2}$

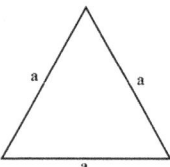

### Trapezoid

$P = a + b + c + d$

$A = \dfrac{a+b}{2} h$

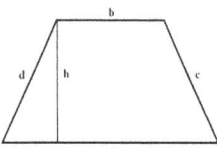

### Circle

$P = 2r\pi$

$A = r^2 \pi$

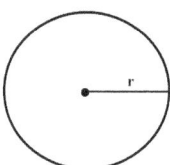

**Area and Volume (3-dimentional shapes)**

To calculate the area of a 3-dimentional shape, we calculate the areas of all sides and then we add them all.

To find the volume of a 3-dimentional shape, we multiply the area of the base (B) and the height (H) of the 3-dimentional shape.

$$V = BH$$

In case of a pyramid and a cone, the volume would be divided by 3.

$$V = BH/3$$

**Example Problems**

**Determine the Surface Area of a 3-D Solid**

Surface Area = 2(Base Area) + (Perimeter) *(Height)

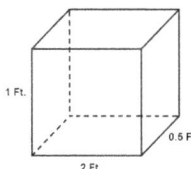

Base Area = 2 ft * 0.5 ft = 1 ft$^2$
Perimeter = 2 ft + 0.5 f t + 2 ft + 0.5 ft  = 5 ft
Height = 1 ft
Surface Area = 2(1 ft$^2$) + (5 ft) * (1 ft) = 2 ft$^2$ + 5 ft$^2$ = 6 ft$^2$

**Determine the Volume of a 3-D Solid**

Volume = (Base Area) * (Height)

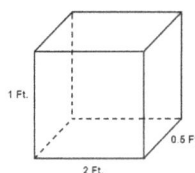

Base Area = 2 ft * 0.5 ft = 1 ft$^2$
Height = 1 ft
Volume = (1 ft$^2$) * (1 ft) = 1 ft$^3$

Here are some of the 3-dimentional shapes with formulas for their area and volume:

## Cuboids

$A = 2(ab + bc + ac)$
$V = abc$

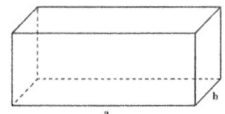

## Cube

$A = 6a^2$
$V = a^3$

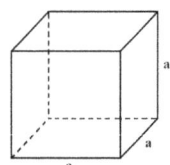

## Pyramid

$A = ab + ah_a + bh_b$
$V = \dfrac{abH}{3}$

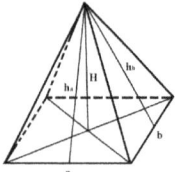

## Cylinder

$A = 2r^2\pi + 2r\pi H$
$V = r^2\pi H$

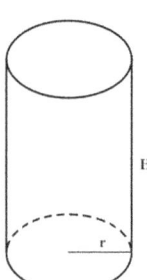

## Cone

$A = (r + s)r\pi$
$V = \dfrac{r^2\pi H}{3}$

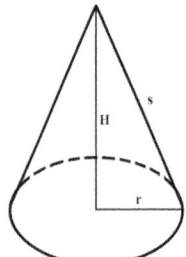

# Area of Complex 2-D and 3-D Shapes

A complex figure is a combination of 2 or more basic shapes.

**Area of a Composite 2-D Shape**

To determine the area of any composite figure, simply add the areas of each component basic figure. Be sure to write you final answer with square units.

**Example Problem**

Determine the area of the given shape.

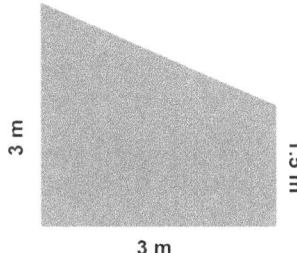

Redraw the original shape as a rectangle and a triangle. Rectangles have opposite sides that are congruent (exactly the same).

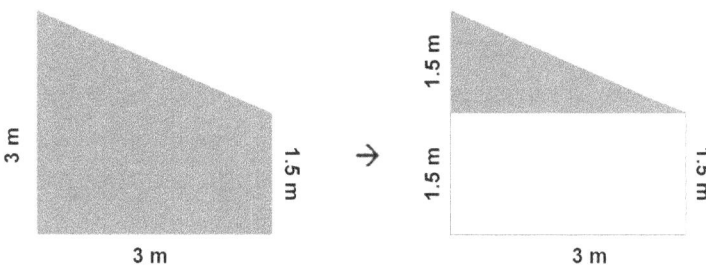

Area $_{Composite}$ = Area $_{Triangle}$ + Area $_{Rectangle}$
Area $_{Triangle}$ = (1/2)(Base)(Height) = (1/2)(3m)(1.5m) = 2.25 m$^2$
Area $_{Rectangle}$ = (Base)(Height) = (3m)(1.5m) = 4.5 m$^2$
Area $_{Composite}$ = (2.25m$^2$) + (4.5m$^2$) = 6.75 m$^2$

**Determine the Surface Area of a Composite 3-D Solid**

To determine the surface area of any composite solid, simply add the surface areas of each component basic solid. You must also subtract the area of any internal face. Be sure to write you final answer with square units.

**Example Problem**

Determine the surface area of the given shape. Leave the final answer in terms of pi. Redraw the original shape as a cylinder and a cone. We will have to subtract the area of the circle where the figures meet from each surface area equation because they are "inside" the solid.

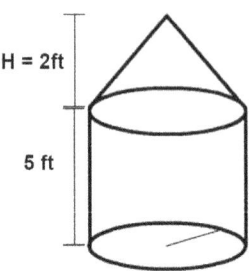

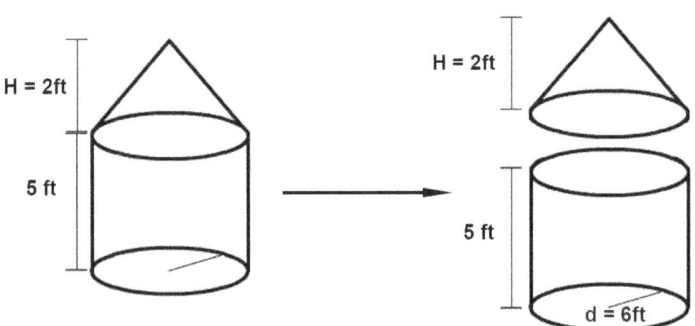

SurfaceArea $_{Composite}$ = S.Area $_{Cone}$ + S.Area $_{Cylinder}$

S.Area $_{Cone}$ = ~~(Base Area)~~+(1/2)(Perimeter)(Height) = (1/2)(dπ)(h) = (1/2)(6π)(2) = 6π ft²

S.Area $_{Cylinder}$ = ~~2~~(Base Area)+(Perimeter)(Height) = (πr²)+(dπ)(h) = (π3²)+(6π)(5) = 39π ft²

S.Area $_{Composite}$ = (6π ft²) + (39π ft²) = 45π ft²

## Pythagorean Geometry

If we have a right triangle ABC, where its sides (legs) are a and b and c is a hypotenuse (the side opposite the right angle), then we can establish a relationship between these sides using the following formula:

$c^2 = a^2 + b^2$

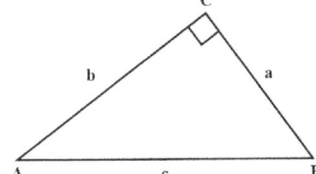

This formula is proven in the Pythagorean Theorem. There are many proofs of this theorem, but we'll look at just one geometrical proof:

If we draw squares on the right triangle's sides, then the area of the hypotenuse square will be equal to the sum of the areas of the squares on the two sides. Since the areas of these squares are a², b² and c², that is how we got the formula above.

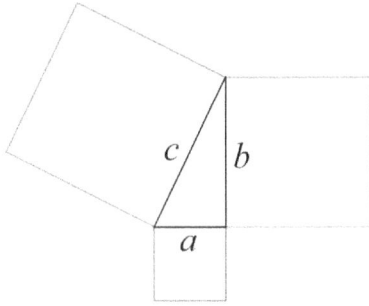

One of the famous right triangles is one with sides 3, 4 and 5. And we can see here that:

3² + 4² = 5²
9 + 16 = 25
25 = 25

**Example Problem:**

The isosceles triangle ABC has a perimeter of 18 centimeters, and the difference between its base and legs is 3 centimeters. Find the height of this triangle.

We write the information we have about triangle ABC and we draw a picture of it for

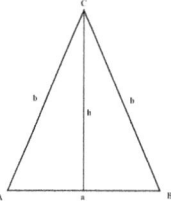

better understanding of the relation between its elements:

P=18 cm
a - b = 3 cm
h=?

We use the formula for the perimeter of the isosceles triangle, since that is what is given to us:

P=a+2b=18 cm

Notice that we have 2 equations with 2 variables, so we can solve it as a system of equations:

a + 2b = 18
a − b = 3 / a + 2b = 18
2a - 2b = 6 / a + 2b + 2a - 2b = 18 + 6
3a = 24
a = 24/3 = 8 cm

Now we go back to find b:
a - b = 3
8 - b = 3
b = 8 - 3
b = 5 cm

Using Pythagorean Theorem, we can find the height using a and b, because the height falls on the side a at the right angle. Notice that height cuts side a exactly in half, and that's why we use in the formula a/2. Here, b is our hypotenuse, so we have:

$b^2 = (a/2)^2 + h^2$
$h^2 = b^2 - (a/2)^2$
$h^2 = 5^2 - (8/2)^2$
$h^2 = 5^2 - (8/2)^2$
$h^2 = 25 - 4^2$
$h^2 = 26 - 16$
$h^2 = 9$
h = 3 cm.

## Adding and Subtracting Polynomials

When we are adding or subtracting 2 or more polynomials, we have to first group the same variables (arguments) that have the same degrees and then add or subtract them. For example, if we have $ax^3$ in one polynomial (where a is some real number), we have to group it with $bx^3$ from the other polynomial (where b is also some real number). Here is one example with adding polynomials:

$(-x^2 + 2x + 3) + (2x^2 + 4x - 5) =$
$-x^2 + 2x + 3 + 2x^2 + 4x - 5 =$
$x^2 + 6x - 2$

We remove the brackets, and since we have a plus in front of every bracket, the signs in the polynomials don't change.
We group variables with the same degrees. We have -1 + 2, which is 1 and that's how we got $x^2$. For the first degree, where we have 2 + 4 which is 6, and the constants (real numbers) where we have 3 - 5 which is -2.

The principle is the same with subtracting, only we have to keep in mind that a minus in front of the polynomial changes all signs in that polynomial. Here is one example:

$(4x^3 - x^2 + 3) - (-3x^2 - 10) =$
$4x^3 - x^2 + 3 + 3x^2 + 10 =$
$4x^3 + 2x^2 + 13$

We remove the brackets, and since we have a minus in front of the second polynomial, all signs in that polynomial change. We have -3 x 2 and with minus in front, it becomes a plus and same goes for -10.

Now we group the variables with same degrees: there is no variable with the third degree in the second polynomial, so we just write 4 x 3. We group other variables the same way as adding polynomials.

## Multiplying and Dividing Polynomials

If we have two polynomials that we need to multiply, then multiply each member of the first polynomial with each member of the second. Let's see in one example how this works:

$(x - 1)(x - 2) = x^2 - 2x - x + 2 = x^2 - 3x + 2$

The first member of the first polynomial is multiplied with the first member of the second polynomial and then with the second member of the second polynomial. Continue the process with the second member of the first polynomial, then simplify.

To multiply more polynomials, multiply the first 2, then multiply that result with next polynomial and so on. Here is one example:

$(1 - x)(2 - x)(3 - x) = (2 - x - 2x + x^2)(3-x)$
$= (2 - 3x + x^2)(3 - x)$
$= 6 - 2x - 9x + 3x^2 + 3x^2 - x^3 = 6 - 11x + 6x^2 - x^3$

## Simplifying Polynomials

Let's say we are given some expression with one or more variables, where we have to add, subtract and multiply polynomials. We do the calculations with variables and constants and then we group the variables with the appropriate degrees. As a result, we would get a polynomial. This process is called simplifying polynomials, where we go from a complex expression to a simple polynomial.

Example:

Simplify the following expression and arrange the degrees from bigger to smaller:

$4 + 3x - 2x^2 + 5x + 6x^3 - 2x^2 + 1 = 6x^3 - 4x^2 + 8x + 5$

We can have more complex expressions such as:

$(x + 5)(1 - x) - (2x - 2) = x - x^2 + 5 - 5x - 2x + 2 = -x^2 - 6x + 7$

Here, first we multiply the polynomials and then we subtract the result and the third polynomial.

## Factoring Polynomials

If we have a polynomial that we want to write as multiplication of a real number and a polynomial or as a multiplication of 2 or more polynomials, then we are dealing with factoring polynomials.

Let's see an example of simple factoring:

$12x^2 + 6x - 4 =$
$2 * 6x^2 + 2 * 3x - 2 * 2 =$
$2(6x^2 + 3x - 2)$

We look at every polynomial member as a product of a real number and a variable. Notice that all real numbers in the polynomial are even, so they have the same number (factor). We pull out that 2 in front of the polynomial, and we write what is left.

What if have a more complex case, where we can't find a factor that is a real number? Here is an example:

$x^2 - 2x + 1 =$
$x^2 - x - x + 1 =$
$x(x - 1) - (x - 1) =$
$(x - 1)(x - 1)$

We can write -2x as –x-x . Now we group first 2 members and we see that they have the same factor x, which we can pull in front of them. For the other 2 members, we pull the minus in front of them, so we can get the same binomial that we got with the first 2 members. Now we have that this binomial is the factor for x(x - 1) and (x - 1).
If we pull x - 1 in front (underlined), from the first member, we are left with x, and from the second we have -1.

That is how we transform a polynomial into a product of 2 polynomials (here binomials).

## Quadratic equations

### A. Factoring

Quadratic equations are called second degree equations, which means that the second degree is the highest degree of the variable that can be found in the quadratic equation. The form of these equations is:

$$ax^2 + bx + c = 0$$

where a, b and c are some real numbers.

One way for solving quadratic equations is the factoring method, where we transform the quadratic equation into a product of 2 or more polynomials. Let's see how that works in one simple example:

$x^2 + 2x = 0$

$x(x + 2) = 0$

$(x = 0) \vee (x + 2 = 0)$

$(x = 0) \vee (x = -2)$

Notice that here we don't have parameter c, but this is still a quadratic equation, because we have the second degree of variable x. Our factor here is x, which we put in front, and we are left with x+2. The equation is equal to 0, so either x or x+2 are 0, or both are 0.
So, our 2 solutions are 0 and -2.

### B. Quadratic formula
If we are unsure how to rewrite quadratic equations so we can solve it using the factoring method, we can use the formula for quadratic equation:

$$x_{1,2} = \frac{-b \pm \sqrt{b^2 - 4ac}}{2a}$$

We write $x_{1,2}$ because it represents 2 solutions of the equation. Here is one example:

$3x^2 - 10x + 3 = 0$

$x_{1,2} = \frac{-b \pm \sqrt{b^2 - 4ac}}{2a}$

$x_{1,2} = \frac{-(-10) \pm \sqrt{(-10)^2 - 4 \cdot 3 \cdot 3}}{2 \cdot 3}$

$x_{1,2} = \frac{10 \pm \sqrt{100 - 36}}{6}$

$x_{1,2} = \frac{10 \pm \sqrt{64}}{6}$

$x_{1,2} = \frac{10 \pm 8}{6}$

$x_1 = \frac{10 + 8}{6} = \frac{18}{6} = 3$

$x_2 = \frac{10 - 8}{6} = \frac{2}{6} = \frac{1}{3}$

We see that a is 3, b is -10 and c is 3.
We use these numbers in the equation and do some calculations.

Notice that we have + and -, so $x_1$ is for + and $x_2$ is for -, and that's how we get 2 solutions.

## Momentum

Momentum can be described as the sum product of the mass of an object and its velocity. This means that momentum measures the force produced by an object's mass and velocity.

The formula for calculating momentum is = Momentum = mass X velocity
Or
P = MV
Where P = momentum, V = velocity and M = mass

Based on the above definition, clearly the momentum of a car and a bicycle both travelling at 20 m/s will not be the same, because although the velocity of the two objects are the same, their mass is different. The car would have greater momentum, due to its larger mass.

Note that:

The SI unit for velocity = m/s
SI unit for Mass = kg
Therefore momentum = kg x m/s and SI unit for momentum is kg x m/s

Momentum must always have a direction and so the final answer must reflect the direction of the momentum or velocity.

Sample questions

1
Find the momentum of a round stone weighing 12.05 kg rolling down a hill at 8m/s.

Formula - P= kg x m/s
= 12.05kg x 8m/s
= 96.4 kg x m/s down hill

Take note that the final answer has the proper SI unit of momentum (kg x m/s) after it and it also mentions the direction of the movement.

2
A cannon ball weighing 35kg is shot from a cannon towards the east at 220mls, calculate the momentum of the cannon ball.

Formula - P= kg x m/s
= 35kg x 220m/s
= 7700 kg x m/s east

# SCIENCE

This section contains a science self-assessment and tutorials. The Tutorials are designed to familiarize general principles and the self-assessment contains general questions similar to the science questions likely to be on the PAX RN exam, but are not intended to be identical to the exam questions. Many Universities recommend that students take an introductory Science course before taking the PAX RN Exam. The tutorials are *not* designed to be a complete science course, and it is assumed that students have some familiarity with Science. If you do not understand parts of the tutorial, or find the tutorial difficult, it is recommended that you seek out additional instruction.

## Tour of the PAX RN Science Content

The PAX RN science section currently has 100 science questions which cover Biology, Chemistry, and Physics. The Physics component is currently being tested and is not given at all institutions. Be sure to check with your school for the exact content of the exam you will be taking. Below is a detailed list of the science topics likely to appear on the PAX RN.

**Biology**

- Cellular processes
- Scientific reasoning and scientific method
- Classification and Taxonomy
- Photosynthesis
- Genetics

**Chemistry**

- Atoms and molecules
- Protons and electrons
- States of matter
- Redox reactions
- Chemical reactions
- Acid and base
- Molarity
- Periodic table

**Physics**

- Potential, mechanical and kinetic energy
- Electricity - currents voltage and resistance
- Ohm's law
- Newton's laws
- Linear and rotational motion

The questions below are not the same as you will find on the PAX RN - that would be too easy! And nobody knows what the questions will be and they change all the time. Mostly the changes consist of substituting new questions for old, but the changes also can be new question formats or styles, changes to the number of questions in each section, changes to the time limits for each section and combing sections. Below are general Science questions that cover the same areas as the PAX RN. So the format and exact wording of the questions may differ slightly, and changes from year to year, if you can answer the questions below, you will have no problem with the Science section of the PAX RN.

## Science Self Assessment

The purpose of the self-assessment is:

- Identify your strengths and weaknesses.
- Develop your personalized study plan (above)
- Get accustomed to the PAX RN format
- Extra practice – the self-assessment is a 3rd test!
- Provide a baseline score for preparing your study schedule.

Since this is a self-assessment, and depending on how confident you are with basic science, timing yourself is optional. The biology, chemistry and optional physics sections have 75 questions to be answered in 75 minutes. The self-assessment has 30 questions, so allow 50 minutes to complete.

Once complete, use the table below to assess you understanding of the content, and prepare your study schedule described in chapter 1.

| 80% - 100% | Excellent – you have mastered the content |
|---|---|
| 60% – 79% | Good. You have a working knowledge. Even though you can just pass this section, you may want to review the tutorials and do some extra practice to see if you can improve your mark. |
| 40% - 59% | Below Average. You do not understand the content.<br><br>Review the tutorials, and retake this quiz again in a few days, before proceeding to the Practice Test Questions. |
| Less than 40% | Poor. You have a very limited understanding of the content.<br><br>Please review the tutorials, and retake this quiz again in a few days, before proceeding to the Practice Test Questions. |

**Science Self Assessment**

1. A B C D
2. A B C D
3. A B C D
4. A B C D
5. A B C D
6. A B C D
7. A B C D
8. A B C D
9. A B C D
10. A B C D
11. A B C D
12. A B C D
13. A B C D
14. A B C D
15. A B C D
16. A B C D
17. A B C D
18. A B C D
19. A B C D
20. A B C D
21. A B C D
22. A B C D
23. A B C D
24. A B C D
25. A B C D
26. A B C D
27. A B C D
28. A B C D
29. A B C D
30. A B C D

# Physics

**1. Which of the following is not true of atomic theory?**

a. Originated 2500 years ago with Greek philosopher, Leucippus and his pupil Democritus

b. Is the field of physics that describes the characteristics and properties of atoms that make up matter.

c. Explains temperature as the momentum of atoms.

d. Explains macroscopic phenomenon through the behavior of microscopic atoms.

**2. Which of these statements about atoms is/are correct?**

a. Atoms are the largest unit of matter that can take part in a chemical reaction.

b. Atoms can be broken down chemically into much simpler forms.

c. Atoms are composed of protons and neutrons in a central nucleus surrounded by electrons.

d. Atoms do not differ in terms of atomic number or atomic mass.

**3. Protons, neutrons, and electrons differ in that:**

a. Protons and neutrons form the nucleus of an atom, while electrons are found in fixed energy levels around the nucleus of the atom.

b. Protons and neutrons are charged particles and electrons are neutral.

c. Protons and neutrons form fixed energy levels around the nucleus of the atom and electrons are located near the surface of the atom.

d. Protons, neutrons and electrons are charged particles.

**4. Newton's laws of motion consist of three physical laws that form the basis for classical mechanics. Which of the following is/are not included in these laws?**

a. Unless acted on by a force, a body at rest stays at rest.

b. Unless acted on by a force, a body in motion will change direction and gradually slow until it eventually stops.

c. To every action, there is an equal and opposite reaction.

d. A body acted on by a force will accelerate in the same direction as the force at a magnitude that is directly proportional to the force.

5. A car starts from a full stop and in 20 seconds is travelling 10/m per second. What is the acceleration?

    a. 0.5 m/sec$^2$

    b. 0.24 m/sec$^2$

    c. 1 m/sec$^2$

    d. 1.5 m/sec$^2$

6. The space station travels 1000 meters in 5 seconds. How fast is it travelling?

    a. 100 meters/second

    b. 200 meters/second

    c. 50 meters/second

    d. 500 meters/second

7. How much force is needed to accelerate a car weighing 2,000 kg, at a rate of 3 m/s$^2$?

    a. 6000 N

    b. 3000 N

    c. 2000 N

    d. 1000 N

8. Protons, neutrons, and electrons differ in that:

    a. Protons and neutrons form the nucleus of an atom, while electrons are found in fixed energy levels around the nucleus of the atom.

    b. Protons and neutrons are charged particles and electrons are neutral.

    c. Protons and neutrons form fixed energy levels around the nucleus of the atom and electrons are located near the surface of the atom.

    d. Protons, neutrons and electrons are charged particles.

## Biology

9. Classification is a grouping of organisms based on similar

    a. Traits and evolutionary histories

    b. Traits and biological histories

    c. Behaviors and evolutionary histories

    d. Traits and evolutionary advancement

**10. A method for categorizing organisms by their biological type is known as:**

   a. Anatomical classification.
   b. Biological classification.
   c. Physical classification.
   d. Cellular classification.

**11. When compared to homologous traits, "analogous" traits refer to ones that:**

   a. Are similar but the similarity does not derive from a common ancestor.
   b. Are similar because they had the same parents.
   c. Are not similar and do not come from a common ancestor.
   d. Are equal.

**12. Which, if any, of the following statements about mitosis are correct?**

   a. Mitosis is the process of cell division by which identical daughter cells are produced.
   b. Following mitosis, new cells contain less DNA than did the original cells.
   c. During mitosis, the chromosome number is doubled.
   d. A and C are correct.

**13. What is a nucleic acid that carries the genetic information in the cell and is capable of self-replication?**

   a. RNA
   b. Triglyceride
   c. DNA
   d. DAR

**14. The segment of a DNA molecule determining the amino acid sequence of protein is known as**

   a. Operator gene
   b. Structural gene
   c. Regulator gene
   d. Modifier gene

**15. Cells that line the inner or outer surfaces of organs or body cavities are often linked together by intimate physical connections. What are these connections?**

    a. Separate desmosomes

    b. Ronofilaments

    c. Tight junctions

    d. Fascia adherenes

**16. Genes control heredity in man and other organisms. These genes are**

    a. A segment of RNA or DNA

    b. A bead like structure on the chromosomes

    c. A protein molecule

    d. A segment of RNA

**17. Who was a 19th century scientist who outlined the original theory of inheritance?**

    a. Albert Einstein

    b. Christian Doppler

    c. Gregor Mendel

    d. Charles Darwin

**18. Describe the science of genetics.**

    a. Is a branch of biology concerned with the study of heredity and variation.

    b. Attempts to explain how characteristics of living organisms are passed on from one generation to the next.

    c. Is a measure of the variety of the of the Earth's animal, plant, and microbial species.

    d. A and B

**19. Describe enzymes**

    a. Most enzymes are proteins that are selective catalysts

    b. Enzymes are catalysts that accelerate metabolic reactions

    c. Enzymes are chemical agents that assist metabolic reactions

    d. Enzymes are biological agents that decrease the rate of reaction

## Chemistry

**20. In the periodic table, elements are arranged in order of their atomic _____, which is the number of _____ found in their nucleus.**

  a. Mass, protons
  b. Number, neutrons
  c. Mass, neutrons
  d. Number, protons

**21. What are the differences, if any, between mixtures and compounds?**

  a. A mixture is homogeneous, and the properties of its components are retained, while a compound is heterogeneous and its properties are distinct from those of the elements combined in its formation.

  b. A mixture is heterogeneous, and the properties of its components are retained, while a compound is homogeneous and its properties are distinct from those of the elements combined in its formation.

  c. A mixture is heterogeneous, and the properties of its components are changed, while a compound is homogeneous and its properties are similar to those of the elements combined in its formation.

  d. A compound is heterogeneous, and the properties of its components are retained, while a mixture is homogeneous and its properties are distinct from those of the elements combined in its formation.

**22. What are the differences, if any, between chemical changes and physical changes?**

  a. During a physical change, some aspect of the physical properties of matter are altered, but the identity of the substance remains constant. Chemical changes involve the alteration of both a substance's composition and structure.

  b. During a chemical change, some aspect of the physical properties of matter are altered, but the identity of the substance remains constant. Physical changes involve the alteration of both a substance's composition and structure.

  c. During a physical change, no aspects of the physical properties of matter are altered, but the identity of the substance remains constant. Chemical changes involve the alteration of both a substance's composition and structure.

  d. There is no substantive difference between chemical and physical changes.

23. A _____ is a process that transforms one set of chemical substances to another; the substances used are known as _____ and those formed are _____.

   a. A chemical change is a process that transforms one set of chemical substances to another; the substances used are known as products and those formed are reactants.

   b. A biological change is a process that transforms one set of chemical substances to another; the substances used are known as reactants and those formed are products.

   c. A chemical change is a process that transforms one set of chemical substances to another; the substances used are known as reactants and those formed are products.

   A chemical variation is a process that transforms one set of chemical substances to another; the substances used are known as reactants and those formed are products.

24. _____ is the most abundant element in the Earth's crust and appears on the Atomic Table as the letter ____.

   a. Nitrogen, N
   b. Oxygen, O
   c. Silicon, Si
   d. Sodium, Na

25. The elements in the periodic table are arranged in

   a. Order of increasing atomic number
   b. Alphabetical order
   c. Order of increasing metallic properties
   d. Order of increasing neutron content

26. The molarity of 5 liters of a salt solution is 0.5 M of salt solution. Calculate the moles of salt in the solution.

   a. 1
   b. 2
   c. 2.5
   d. 3

## Scientific Reasoning

**27. In science, _____ is defined as a difference between the desired and actual performance or behavior of a system or object.**

    a. Accuracy

    b. Uncertainty

    c. Error

    d. Mistake

**28. When employing the scientific method of research, the researcher follows these steps:**

    a. Define the question, make observations, offer a possible explanation, perform an experiment, analyze data, draw conclusions.

    b. Make observations, offer a possible explanation, define the question, perform an experiment, analyze, draw conclusions.

    c. Perform an experiment, make observations, define the question, offer a possible explanation, analyze the data, draw conclusions.

    d. Make observations, define the question, offer a possible explanation, perform an experiment, analyze data, draw conclusions.

**29. What is the principle that generally advises choosing the competing hypothesis that makes the fewest new assumptions, when the hypotheses are equal in other respects?**

    a. Hickam's Dictum

    b. Boyle's Law

    c. Dalton's Law

    d. Occam's Razor

**30. A _____ _____ is a statistic used as a measure of the dispersion or variation in a distribution.**

    a. Normal distribution

    b. Range

    c. Outlier

    d. Standard deviation

# Answer Key

## 1. C
Answer c is incorrect because atomic theory explains temperature as the motion of atoms (faster = hotter), not the momentum. The momentum of atoms explains the outward pressure that they exert.

## 2. C
The only correct statement about atoms is they "Are composed of protons and neutrons in a central nucleus surrounded by electrons."

## 3. A
Protons and neutrons form the nucleus of an atom, while electrons are found infixed energy levels around the nucleus of the atom.

## 4. B
Unless acted on by a force, a body in motion will change direction and gradually slow until it eventually stops.

This answer is related to Newton's 1st law of motion that states that, unless acted on by a force, a body at rest stays at rest, and a moving body continues moving at the same speed in a straight line.

## 5. A
The formula for acceleration = $A = (V_f - V_0)/t$
so $A = (10 \text{ m/sec} - 0 \text{ m/sec})/20 \text{ sec} = 0.5 \text{ m/sec}^2$

## 6. B
Speed = (total distance traveled)/(total time taken)
1000/5 = 200 meters per second

## 7. A
Force = Mass times Acceleration Measured in Newtons.
$F = 2000 \text{ kg} \times 3 \text{ m/sec}^2 = 6000 \text{ N}$

## 8. A
Protons and neutrons form the nucleus of an atom, while electrons are found infixed energy levels around the nucleus of the atom.

# Biology

## 9. A
Classification is a grouping of organisms based on similar traits and evolutionary histories.

**Note:** Taxonomy and systematics are the two sciences that attempt to classify living things. Taxonomy assigns organisms to groups based on their characteristics. In modern systematics, the placement of organisms into groups is based on evolutionary relationships.

**10. B**

Biological classification. Classification is more a matter of convenience; in reality, there are many times when the various classifications tend to blur into each other.

**11. A**

Analogous traits are similar but the similarity does not derive from a common ancestor.

**12. A and C are correct.**

    a. Mitosis is the process of cell division by which identical daughter cells are produced.

    c. During mitosis, the chromosome number is doubled.

**13. C**

DNA is a nucleic acid that carries the genetic information in the cell and is capable of self-replication.

**14. B**

A structural gene is the segment of a DNA molecule determining the amino acid sequence of protein. DNA is a nucleic acid that contains the genetic instructions used in the development and functioning of all known living organisms (with the exception of RNA viruses). The DNA segments that carry this genetic information are called genes but other DNA sequences have structural purposes or are involved in regulating the use of this genetic information. Along with RNA and proteins DNA is one of the three major macromolecules that are essential for all known forms of life.

**15. C**

Tight junctions are the areas of two cells with membranes join an impermeable barrier to fluid. This type of junction is only found in vertebrates.

**16. A**

Genes are made from a long molecule called DNA which is copied and inherited across generations. DNA is made of simple units that line up in a particular order within this large molecule. The order of these units carries genetic information similar to how the order of letters on a page carries information. The language used by DNA is called the genetic code which lets organisms read the information in the genes. This information is instructions for constructing and operating a living organism.

**17. C**

Gregor Mendel was a 19th century scientist who outlined the original theory of inheritance.

**18. D**

A and B describe genetics.

    a. Is a branch of biology concerned with the study of heredity and variation.

    b. Attempts to explain how characteristics of living organisms are passed on from one generation to the next.

### 19. A
Most enzymes are proteins that are selective catalysts

## Chemistry

### 20. D
In the Periodic Table, elements are arranged in order of their atomic number, which is the number of protons found in their nucleus.

### 21. B
A mixture is heterogeneous, and the properties of its components are retained, while a compound is homogeneous and its properties are distinct from those of the elements combined in its formation.

### 22. A
During a physical change, some aspect of the physical properties of matter are altered, but the identity of the substance remains constant. Chemical changes involve the alteration of both a substance's composition and structure.

### 23. C
A chemical change is a process that transforms one set of chemical substances to another; the substances used are known as reactants and those formed are products.

### 24. B
Oxygen is the most abundant element in the Earth's crust and appears on the Atomic Table as the letter O.

### 25. A
The periodic table of the chemical elements (also known as the periodic table or periodic table of the elements) is a tabular display of the 118 known chemical elements organized by selected properties of their atomic structures. Elements are presented by increasing atomic number, the number of protons in an atom's atomic nucleus.

### 26. C
Moles of solute = ? or X
Solutions liters = 5 liters
Molarity of solution = 0.5 M

Therefore:   X moles/5 liters of solution = 0.5 or X/5 = 0.5
So X = 5/0.5
X = 2.5

## Scientific Method and Reasoning

### 27. C
In science, Error is a difference between the desired and actual performance or behavior of a system or object.

**28. A**

When employing the scientific method of research, the researcher follows these steps: define the question, make observations, offer a possible explanation, perform an experiment, analyze data, draw conclusions.

**29. D**

Occam's Razor is a principle that generally advises choosing the competing hypothesis that makes the fewest new assumptions, when the hypotheses are equal in other respects.

**30. D**

A Standard deviation is a statistic used as a measure of the dispersion or variation in a distribution.

## Science Tutorials

## Scientific Method

**The scientific method is a set of steps that allow people who ask "how" and "why" questions about the world to go about finding valid answers that accurately reflect reality.**

> WIthout the scientific method, people would have no valid method for drawing quantifiable and accurate information about the world.

**There are four primary steps to the scientific method:**

1. Analyzing an aspect of reality and asking "how" or "why" it works or exists
2. Forming a hypothesis that explains "how" or "why"
3. Making a prediction about the sort of things that would happen if the hypothesis were true
4. Performing an experiment to test your prediction.

> These steps vary somewhat depending on the field of science you happen to be studying. (In astronomy, for instance, experiments are generally eschewed in favor of observational evidence confirming that predictions are true.) But for the most part, this is the model scientists follow.

**Observation and Analysis**

**The first step in the scientific method requires you to determine what it is about reality that you want to explore.**

> You might notice that your friends who eat regular servings of fruits and vegetables are healthier and more athletic than your friends who live off red meat and meals covered in cheese and gravy. This is an observation and, noting it, you are likely to ask yourself "why" it seems to be true. At this stage of the scientific method, scientists will often do research to see if anyone else has explored similar observations and analyze what other people's findings have been. This is an important step not only because it shows what others have found to be true about their observation, but because it can show what others have found to be false, which can be equally valuable.

**Hypothesis**

**After making your observation and doing some research, you can form your hypothesis. A hypothesis is an idea you formulate based on the evidence you have already gathered about "how" your observation relates to reality.**

Using the example of your friends' diets, you may have found research discussing vitamin levels in fruits and vegetables and how certain vitamins will affect a person's health and athleticism. This research may lead you to hypothesize that the foods your healthy friends are eating contain specific types of vitamins, and it is the vitamins making them healthy. Just as important, however, is applying research that shows hypotheses that were later proven wrong. Scientists need to know this information, too, as it can help keep them from making errors in their thinking. For instance, you could come across a research paper in which someone hypothesized that the sugars in fruits and vegetables gave people more energy, which then helped them be more athletic. If the paper were to go onto explain that no such link was found, and that the protein and carbohydrates in meat and gravy contained far more energy than the sugar, you would know that this hypothesis was wrong and that there was no need for you to waste time exploring it.

**Prediction**

**The third step in the scientific method is making a prediction based on your hypothesis.**

Forming predictions is vital to the scientific method, because, if your prediction turns out to be correct, it will demonstrate that your hypothesis can accurately explain some aspect of the world. This is important because one aspect of the scientific method is its ability to prove objectively that your way of understanding the world is valid. We can take the simple example of a car that will not start. If you notice the fuel gauge is pointing towards empty, you can announce your prediction to the other passengers that a careful test of the gas tank will show the car has no fuel. While this seems obvious, it is still important to note since a prediction like this is the only way to really *prove* to your friends that you understand how a fuel gauge works and what it means.

In the same way, a prediction made by a hypothesis is the only way to show that it represents reality. For instance, based on your vitamin hypothesis you may predict people can be healthy and athletic while eating whatever they want, as long as they take vitamin supplements. If this prediction ends being true, it will show that it is in fact the vitamins, and only the vitamins, in fruits and vegetables that make people healthy and athletic. It will prove that your hypothesis shows how vitamins work.

**Experiment**

**The final step is to perform an experiment that tests your prediction.**
You may decide to separate your healthy friends into three groups, give one group vitamin supplements and prohibit them from eating vegetables, give another fake supplements and prohibit them from eating vegetables and have the third act normally as the control group. It is always important to have a control group so you have someone acting "normally" to compare your results against. If this experiment shows the real supplement group and the control group maintaining the same level of health and athleticism, while the fake supplement group grows weak and sickly, you will know your hypothesis is true. If, on the other hand, you get unexpected results, you will need to go back to step one, analyze your results, make new observations and try again with a different hypothesis.

Any hypothesis that cannot be confirmed with experiment (or in the case of fields such as astronomy, with observation) cannot be considered true and must be altered or abandoned. It is in this stage where scientists—being humans, with human beliefs and prejudices—are most likely to abandon the scientific method. If an experiment or observation gives a scientist results that he or she does not like, the scientist may be inclined to ignore the results rather than reexamine the hypothesis. This was the case for nearly a thousand years in astronomy with astronomers attempting to form accurate models of the solar system based on circular orbits of the planets and on Earth being in the center. For philosophical reasons the ancients believed circles were "perfect" and that the Earth was "important," so no model that had the correct elliptical orbits or the sun properly in the center was accepted until the 16$^{th}$ century, even though those models more accurately described all astronomers' observations.

# Cell Biology

**Cell biology (formerly cytology, from the Greek kytos, "contain") is a scientific discipline that studies cells – their physiological properties, their structure, the organelles they contain, interactions with their environment, their life cycle, division and death.**

This is done both on a microscopic and molecular level. Cell biology research encompasses both the great diversity of single-celled organisms like bacteria and protozoa, as well as the many specialized cells in multicellular organisms such as humans.

**Knowing the components of cells and how cells work is fundamental to all biological sciences.**

Appreciating the similarities and differences between cell types is particularly important to the fields of cell and molecular biology as well as to biomedical fields such as cancer research and developmental biology. These fundamental similarities and differences provide a unifying theme, sometimes allowing the principles learned from studying one cell type to be extrapolated and generalized to other cell types. Therefore, research in cell biology is closely related to genetics, biochemistry, molecular biology, immunology, and developmental biology.

**Each type of protein is usually sent to a particular part of the cell.**

An important part of cell biology is the investigation of molecular mechanisms by which proteins are moved to different places inside cells or secreted from cells.

**Processes – Movement of Proteins**

**Most proteins are synthesized by ribosomes in the rough endoplasmic reticulum.**

Ribosomes contain the nucleic acid RNA, which assembles and joins amino acids to make proteins. They can be found alone or in groups within the cytoplasm as well as on the RER.

**This process is known as protein biosynthesis.**

Biosynthesis (also called biogenesis) is an enzyme-catalysed process in cells of living organisms by which substrates are converted to more complex products (also simply known as protein translation). Some proteins, such as those to be incorporated in membranes (known as membrane proteins), are transported into the "rough" endoplasmic reticulum (ER) during synthesis. This process can be followed by transportation and processing in the Golgi apparatus.

**The Golgi apparatus is a large organelle that processes proteins and prepares them for use both inside and outside the cell.**

The Golgi apparatus is somewhat like a post office. It receives items (proteins from the ER), packages and labels them, and then sends them on to their destinations (to different parts of the cell or to the cell membrane for transport out of the cell). From the Golgi, membrane proteins can move to the plasma membrane, to other sub-cellular compartments, or they can be secreted from the cell.

**The ER and Golgi can be thought of as the "membrane protein synthesis compartment" and the "membrane protein processing compartment," respectively.**

There is a semi-constant flux of proteins through these compartments. ER and Golgi-resident proteins associate with other proteins but remain in their respective compartments. Other proteins "flow" through the ER and Golgi to the plasma membrane. Motor proteins transport membrane protein-containing vesicles along cytoskeletal tracks to distant parts of cells such as axon terminals.

**Some proteins that are made in the cytoplasm contain structural features that target them for transport into mitochondria or the nucleus.**

Some mitochondrial proteins are made inside mitochondria and are coded for by mitochondrial DNA. In plants, chloroplasts also make some cell proteins.

Extracellular and cell surface proteins destined to be degraded can move back into intracellular compartments upon being incorporated into endocytosed vesicles some of which fuse with lysosomes where the proteins are broken down to their individual amino acids. The degradation of some membrane proteins begins while still at the cell surface when they are separated by secretases. Proteins that function in the cytoplasm are often degraded by proteasomes.

**Other cellular processes**

**Active and Passive transport** - Movement of molecules into and out of cells.
**Autophagy** - The process whereby cells "eat" their own internal components or microbial invaders.
**Adhesion** - Holding together cells and tissues.
**Reproduction** - Made possible by the combination of sperm made in the testiculi (contained in some male cells' nuclei) and the egg made in the ovary (contained in the nucleus of a female cell). When the sperm breaks through the hard outer shell of the egg a new cell embryo is formed, which, in humans, grows to full size in 9 months.
**Cell movement** - Chemotaxis, Contraction, cilia and flagella.
**Cell signalling** - Regulation of cell behavior by signals from outside.
**DNA repair and Cell death**
**Metabolism** - Glycolysis, respiration, Photosynthesis
**Transcription and mRNA splicing** - gene expression.

**Internal cellular structures**

**Cytoplasm** - contents of the main fluid-filled space inside cells
**Chloroplast** - organelle for photosynthesis
**Cilia** - motile microtubule containing structures of eukaryotes
**Cytoskeleton** - protein filaments
**Endoplasmic reticulum** - major site of protein synthesis
**Golgi apparatus** - site of protein glycosylation in the endomembrane system
**Flagella** - motile structures of bacteria, archaea and eukaryotes
**Lysosome** - breaks down cellular waste products and debris
**Nucleus** - holds DNA of eukaryotic cells and controls cellular activities
**Ribosome** - RNA and protein complex required for protein synthesis in cells

# Chromosomes, genes, proteins, RNA and DNA

The concepts of genes, chromosomes, proteins, RNA and DNA are all interrelated genetic terms. Chromosomes are made up of genes, the DNA contains the chromosomes and the RNA interprets and implements the information in the RNA. Here is a break down of each of them.

## Proteins

Proteins are biological molecules that are made up of a chain or chains of amino acids. Proteins play many very vital roles in living organisms. Protein is essential for the performance of many bodily functions such as replicating DNA, transporting nutrients and molecules within the body, responding to stimuli, and acting as a catalyst for metabolic reactions within the living organism, among other things. There are different types of proteins and they play various roles. The difference in proteins would be determined by their unique arrangement or sequence of amino acids.

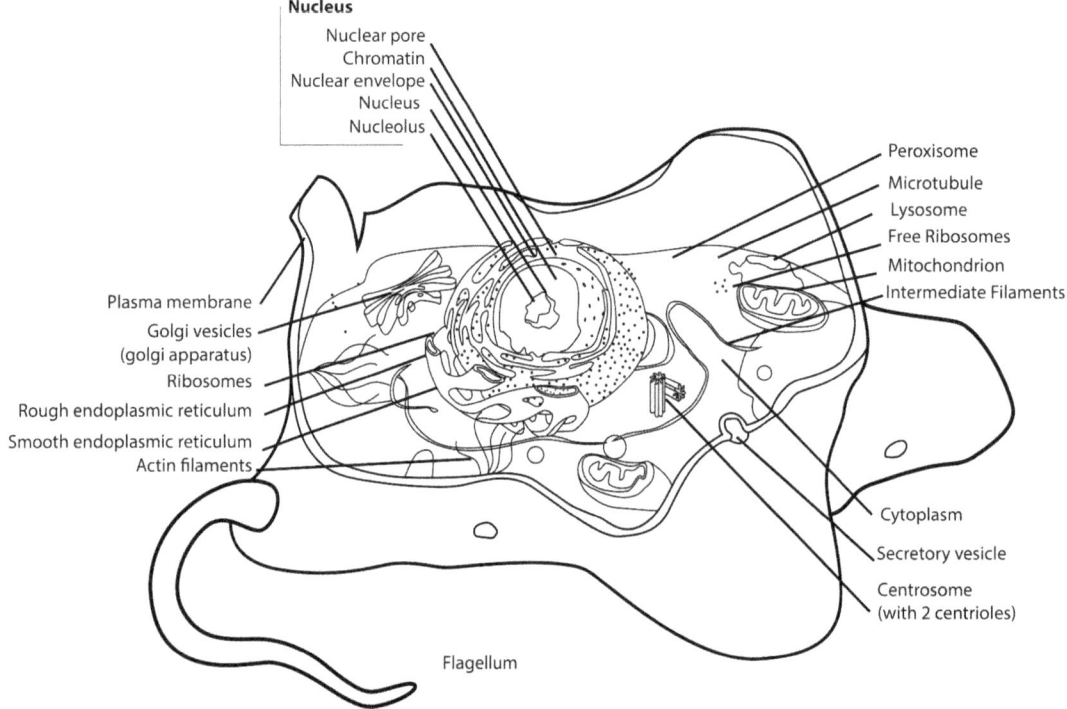

## Genes

A gene is the molecular hereditary unity of an organism and a small part of the chromosome. It is the term used to describe a portion of RNA or DNA code that performs a particular function in the organism. Genes are essential to life because they specify the functions of all proteins and RNA chains. Genes contain the information to maintain and build the cells in the organism and also contain genetic information that would be passed onto the offspring.

Genes hold the information for biological traits and functions some of which can clearly be seen and some of which are hidden. For example, the information contained in specific genes determines factors such as eye color, hair color, number of limbs, height and so on. Some traits such as blood type and the thousands of metabolic reactions and biochemical process that take place in the body to sustain life are defined unseen by the genes.

A gene is set of basic instruction embedded on a sequence of nucleic acids. The gene is a locatable region of the DNA genome sequence that correspond to a unit of inheritance and associated with a particular body function or set of functions.

## Chromosomes

The chromosome is a piece of the DNA containing several genes. The chromosome is an organized part of the DNA. It is a single piece of coiled DNA. The chromosome contains several genes, DNA-bound proteins, nucleotide sequences and regulatory elements. The DNA-bound proteins help to hold the DNA together and regulate its functions.

Since the chromosomes contain the genes, they contain almost all the genetic information of the organism. Chromosomes differ from one organism to another. The DNA molecule could be linear or circular. The chromosome can contain from 100,000 to over 3 million nucleotides in one long chain depending on the organism. Cells with defined nuclei (eukaryotic cells) usually have large linear shaped chromosomes. Cells without clearly defined nuclei (prokaryotic cells) usually have smaller sized circular chromosomes.

Chromosomes are essential in the process of cell division. In mitosis cell division, the chromosomes have to be replicated and then divided among the two resulting daughter cells. This ensures that the resulting two daughter cells are genetically identical to the original mother cell.

## DNA

DNA or Deoxyribonucleic acid is an essential component of life. It has been described as the blueprint of a living organism. It contains vital genetic information and instructions that are required for the proper functioning and development of all types and forms of living organisms and even viruses. DNA, proteins and RNA are the three most important macro-molecules that are essential for any form of life.

The genetic information contained in the DNA is encoded as a sequence of nucleotides known as G, A, and C. With G being guanine, A, adenine, T, thymine and C cytosine. These nucleotides are arranged as DNA molecules in a double-stranded helix. The strands run in opposite directions and are thus anti-parallel. The DNA contains long structures known as chromosomes.

## RNA

RNA or Ribonucleic acids are large biological molecules that perform the important roles of decoding, coding, regulating and expressing the genes and the information contained within them. RNA, DNA and proteins are three essential components for all form of life. The RNA is also composed of nucleotides, but unlike the DNA that is double stranded, the RNA is single stranded.

In organisms, some RNA components serve as messengers to convey genetic information to direct the synthesis or use of specific proteins for specific purposes. RNA is essential for the proper carrying out of the information contained in the DNA genes. RNA plays important roles within the cell such as helping to catalyze biological reactions sense and communicate cellular signals and control gene expressions. RNA is also essential for protein synthesis.

## Mitosis and Meiosis

**Meiosis and mitosis are two types of cellular division that play an important role in cell reproduction and the maintenance of tissues.**

> The cell is the basic functional unit of living organisms. It is made up of a collection of organelles and other cell matter dispersed within the cell membrane. For new cells to form, existing cells divide through the process of meiosis or mitosis, depending on the type of cell and reason for division.

**Mitosis refers to the division of a cell into two identical cells.**

> The original cell goes through a process of duplication of its genetic material and then equally divides its contents into two new daughter cells. The process of mitosis goes through several stages until the two cells segregate to form two distinct but genetically identical cells.

**Mitosis cell division**

> During mitosis the cell divides its nucleus and then separates its organelles and chromosomes into two identical parts. The mother cell then divides into two genetically identical cells with equal parts of the cellular contents. The nuclei, cell membrane, organelles and cytoplasm of the cell would be shared between the two new cells.

Mitosis cell division is a complex and fast process. The process takes place in stages with each stage comprising of a set of activities that leads to the next set. The stages of mitosis are Prophase, Prometaphase, Metaphase, Anaphase and Telophase. Mitosis occurs in some unicellular organisms and within animal and human cells. Unicellular organisms use mitosis to reproduce their like and within animal and humans, mitosis is used to replace cells and repair tissues.

## Meiosis

**Meiosis occurs when one cell from the male and one from the female combine or fuses to form one diploid cell, which then splits to form four haploid cells.**

The diploid cell contains copies of the chromosome and genetic information from both parents. The resulting four haploid cells will contain a copy of each chromosome.

Each chromosome in the four cells will contain a unique blend of the paternal and maternal genetic information, which makes it possible for the offspring to share some genetic resemblance to both parents while remaining genetically distinct from both of them. This nature of meiosis cell division is what accounts for the genetic diversity that is available today as each offspring DNA is a unique blend of its maternal and paternal genetic DNA.

**Mitosis and meiosis have some similarities in that they are both types of cell division among living organisms.**

There is however still some differences among them. For example, mitosis occurs within a cell with no interactions with other cells. The individual cell simply divides and produces two genetically identical cells. With meiosis, the process involves two cells from both the male and female in a form sexual reproduction. The resultant cells are four cells that are genetically different from their parents. Oscar Hertwig discovered meiosis and Walther Flemming discovered mitosis.

## Phenotypes and Genotypes

The terms "phenotype" and "genotype" were first introduced in 1911 by Wilhelm Johannsen.

**The term genotype refers to the genes of an organism that contains its complete hereditary information.**
**Phenotype refers to the actual observed properties of the organism.**

Phenotypes deal with morphology, behavior and development. The distinction between genotypes and phenotypes is a very important fundamental aspect in the study of hereditary traits.

To explain the differences between the two concepts, one may look at genotypes as the inherited information about an organism. It is the genetic makeup of the traits, features and characteristics of the organism. Phenotype on the other hand defines the way that the information as spelled out by the genes is represented. Phenotypes deal with the actual observable development and behavior.

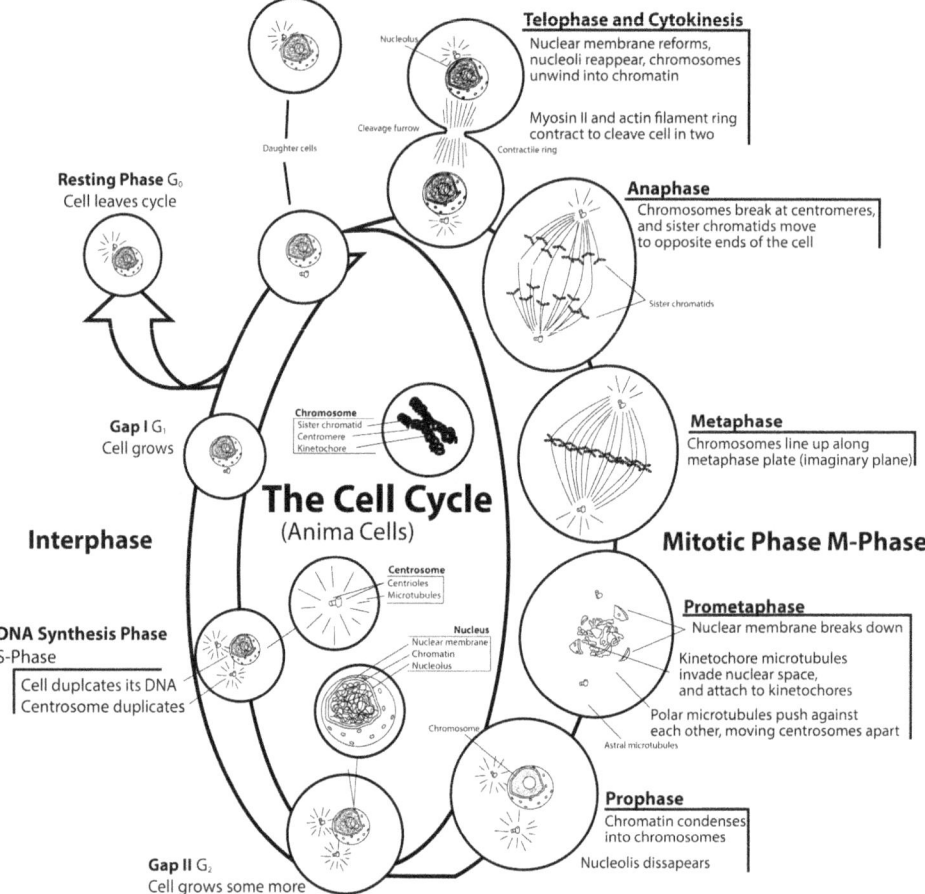

**A small or even minute difference in the genes of two organisms would mean that the two organisms have different genotypes.**

Genes are hereditary and the genetic information contained is passed down from parents under control of specific molecular mechanisms. The genes or genetic information effects or controls the representation of the phenotype.

The genes define the trait or feature of the organism while the phenotype is the observable demonstration or expression of that trait. For example, if a mouse has a white color, it can be said that the genes defines that the mouse would be white and the phenotype is the white color that is observable. The genotype determines the phenotype, but the phenotype is also affected by external factors such as environmental factors.

**A set of genotypes mapped to a set of phenotypes are called a genotype-phenotype map.**

The genotype is the largest influencer of an organism's phenotype, but is not the only influencing factor. That is why two identical twins that share the same genotype would still not have the same phenotypes. They may share identical genomes and their phenotype may even be quite similar, but it cannot be the same. That is why parents and close fiends would always be able to tell them apart. This is because their phenotype or the representation or expression of their genetic makeup as contained in their genotype would not be the same.

The term phenotype plasticity is used to describe the extent to which the genotype of an organism determines its phenotype.

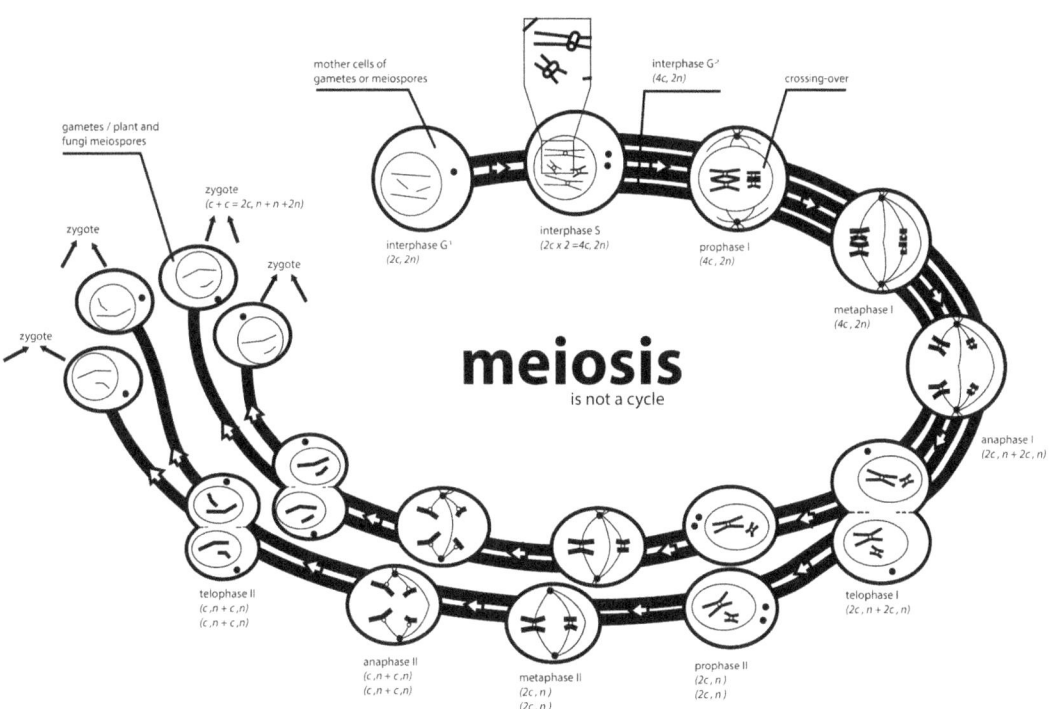

**An organism with weak or little phenotype plasticity would be highly determined more by its genotype and less by environmental factors.**

An organism with high phenotype plasticity would have its phenotype more affected by environmental factors than by its genotype. A good example of an organism with high plasticity whose phenotype is more dependant on its environment than its genotype is the larval newt. The larvae would grow larger sized tails and heads relative to their body size when it notices the presence of their natural predators, i.e., the dragonfly.

**Phenotype canalization is a term used to describe the extent that an organism's phenotype draws conclusions about the organism's genotype.**

An organism with a canalized phenotype would be rarely affected by changes in its genotypes. If canalization is absent, very minor changes in the genome would result in immediate changes in the resulting phenotype.

## Heredity: Genes and Mutation

**All of the genetic material that tells our cells what jobs they hold is stored in our DNA (deoxyribonucleic acid). When complex creatures such as humans reproduce, our DNA is copied and combined with our mate's DNA to create a new genetic sequence for our offspring.**

This information is stored in our genes and encoded in DNA base pairs through different combinations of the chemical groupings adenine and thymine (represented by A and T) and guanine and cytosine (represented by G and C). Each gene covers a small portion of our DNA and is responsible for creating the protein that section of DNA holds instructions for.

**Genes contain two alleles, one from each of our parents. When we reproduce we will transfer one, and only one, of each allele to our children.**

Alleles can be either dominant or recessive, and by combining the pairs of alleles we get from our parents, we can determine what our genes say we should be like. This genetic description of ourselves is known as our genotype. Genotype is our exact genetic makeup, and it determines our physical characteristics such as basic hair, eye and skin color. Related to the genotype is our phenotype, which describes the characteristics we display when our genes interact with the environment. For example, skin color is determined by a person's genotype, but the effect the sun has on skin—does the person tan, freckle, burn or even come away without any noticeable effect at all?—is an expression of phenotype.

**Under normal circumstances people's genes will transfer directly from their parents following Mendel's Laws of Inheritance. Errors are common though.**

DNA reproduction, however, is not necessarily a flawless process. Errors can develop either at random or due to outside influences such as radiation or chemicals in the environment. These errors, when related to heredity are called de novo mutations; they occur during embryonic development. Some mutations have no effect at all on the person's genetic makeup, but others can alter the way genes express themselves. Whether this is a good thing or not depends entirely on what genes are altered in what ways. Some mutations can cause children to be born sick or to have a higher susceptibility to disease by changing the types of proteins that their genes produce, or even by stopping certain proteins from being produced all together. Others, though, can be an improvement to the child's genetic structure. It is important to remember that the entire process of evolution is based on how random mutations throughout history have affected an individual's ability to interact with the environment.

**Several notable examples of beneficial mutations stemming from natural selection can be seen in bubonic plague resistant European populations and malaria resistant African populations.**

Both groups have genes built from specific alleles that create disease blocking proteins. (The CCR5 protein in people of European descent blocks the plague—and HIV sometimes—and the sickle cell protein in people of African descent blocks malaria.) These genes are widespread throughout their respective populations as a result of natural selection, which killed those who lived in these groups' ancestral regions but who did not possess the mutation. Had these diseases never existed, the mutations would have been considered neutral, providing no benefit yet causing no harm.

**There are several ways that errors in DNA reproduction can cause mutations.**

Chemicals can be inserted into, or deleted from base pairs, causing the chemical composition of the pairs to change and, thus, changing the alleles of the gene represented by those pairs. A portion of the DNA strand may also duplicate itself, or it may shift itself, causing the half of the base pair on one side of the DNA strand to link to the wrong half on the other side.

## Heredity: Mendelian Inheritance

**The father of genetics was a 19th century Austrian monk named Gregor Johann Mendel who became famous for his work crossbreeding peas in the garden of his monastery.**

Aside from his life as a monk, Mendel was a highly educated physicist, studying first at the University of Olomouc (in the modern day Czech Republic) and later at the University of Vienna.

**Mendel's work with peas revolutionized the scientific understanding of heredity and yielded two important laws: the Law of Segregation and the Law of Independ-**

ent Assortment. To better understand these laws, however, we first need to look at the work of another geneticist, Reginald Punnett.

In 1900 while Punnett was doing his graduate work at the University of Cambridge in England, Gregor Mendel's work on genetics, which did not receive much attention during his lifetime, was being rediscovered. Punnett became an early follower of Mendelian genetics and developed the Punnett square as a means to organize the assortment of inherited alleles as Mendel described them. A Punnett square is simply a box with several squares drawn inside it and with the allele for a particular gene from each parent listed on either the top or the side. Each square shows a possible genotype (or set of alleles that define the gene) that can be inherited by the offspring of those parents. We will see Punnett squares as we explain Mendel's laws.

## Law of Segregation

**Mendel's Law of Segregation says that only half of the alleles of each parent's genes are transferred to their offspring, with the other half coming from the other parent.**

Each gene contains two alleles. For instance a gene for trait 'A' could contain the alleles AA, Aa or aa, with the 'A' being the dominant form of the allele and 'a' being the recessive form. (Offspring with one or more dominant alleles exhibit the trait; offspring with only recessive forms do not.) The Law of Segregation says that one allele will come from one parent, and one will come from the other, and it is the parent's combined genetic makeup (rather than one parent's particular genotype) that will determine the genes of their offspring.

Mendel also showed that the probability a certain trait would spread from parents to children was 3:1, if both parents had one dominant and one recessive form of the gene, also known has having heterozygous alleles. (Having two of the same alleles—AA or aa—is homozygous.)

### Punnett squares

The Punnett square below represents the possible children born to two parents with Aa alleles expressing the 'A' gene.

|   | **A** | a |
|---|---|---|
| **A** | **AA** | **Aa** |
| a | **Aa** | aa |

The three genes in bold, with at least one capital letter (AA, Aa and the other Aa), represent cases in which the presence of at least one dominant allele will cause the trait to manifest in the offspring. The remaining one (aa) represents the one case where the child does not manifest the trait even though both his or her parents do. (This could be the one brunette in a family of redheads, for instance.) Provided both parents have one dominant and one recessive allele, the distribution will always be 3:1.

**Law of Independent Assortment**

**Mendel's second law, the Law of Independent Assortment, shows that the alleles of multiple genes will mix independently.**

When two separate genotypes are tracked, the genes will produce 16 separate possible combinations spread out in a 9:3:3:1 ratio. This is also known as a di-hybrid cross, while dealing with a single set of alleles is a monohybrid cross.

We can demonstrate this by assuming that we have a male and a female each with heterozygous alleles making them blond and tall. We can represent this with the genotypes BbTt in each. We should also assume that a 'bb' genotype would give someone brown hair and 'tt' would make them short. Since the Law of Independent Assortment says that each allele will mix independently, we end with four combinations of genotype that each parent can pass on: BT, Bt, bT and bt. These can then be mapped in a slightly larger Punnett square that looks like this:

|    | BT | Bt | bT | bt |
|----|----|----|----|----|
| BT | **BBTT** | **BBTt** | **BbTT** | **BbTt** |
| Bt | **BBTt** | **BBtt** | **BbTt** | **Bbtt** |
| bT | **BbTT** | **BbTt** | bbTT | bbTt |
| bt | **BbTt** | **Bbtt** | bbTt | bbtt |

This is the distribution of the tall, blond couple's possible children. Nine would also be tall and blond, three would be short and blond, three would be tall and brunette, and one would be short and brunette. This follows perfectly the 9:3:3:1 ratio set out by Mendel.

# Classification

**Classification**

**Taxonomic classification is the primary method of organizing the Earth's biology. Taxonomy means,**

    **1. The classification of organisms in an ordered system that indicates natural relationships.**
    **2. The science, laws, or principles of classification**

The earliest form of classification that bears any resemblance to the current system can be traced back to ancient Greece with Aristotle's organization of animals based on reproduction.

**The classification into kingdoms (animal, mineral and vegetable) was developed by Carolus Linnaeus.**

The true father of modern taxonomical classification, however, is Carolus Linnaeus, who in the early 18th century developed a system of kingdoms that separated life into the categories animal, mineral and vegetable. Although Linnaeus's work lacked what would today be considered essential technologies (such as microscopes capable of imaging bacteria) and theories (such as evolution), much of his system has survived in modern classification.

**Charles Darwin's theory of evolution was an important factor in taxonomic classification.**

With Charles Darwin's publication of On the Origin of Species in 1859 the evolutionary process became a major factor in taxonomic classification. For the first time biology could be classified by grouping the direct descendants of common ancestors rather than just grouping creatures with similar characteristics.

**The main classifications are, domain, kingdom, phylum, class, order, family, genus and species.**

Today, most scientists accept a hierarchical structuring of biology that goes from general, or large, to specific: domain, kingdom, phylum, class, order, family, genus and species. (There are sometimes smaller subcategories such as superfamily, subfamily, tribe and subspecies listed, but these are the primary eight categories.) Domain is the newest of these and is split into three primary groups: Bacteria, Archaea and Eukarya.
Each of these domains is split again with Bacteria splitting into the Kingdom Bacteria, Archaea splitting into the Kingdom Archaea and Eukarya splitting into the four kingdoms of Protista, Plantae, Fungi and finally our kingdom, Animalia. The Domain Eukarya splits so many times because eukaryotic cells are highly complex, containing such important features as cell walls and nuclei. As a result of this complexity, eukaryotic cells have gone through a much more diverse evolutionary process than prokaryotic cells such as bacteria and archaea, and thus Eukarya make up all complex life on Earth.

**Each Kingdom has a huge number of organisms. Bacteria and Archaea (single celled organisms).**

Within each of the kingdoms the number of creatures is far too many to list. It is estimated that there could be as many as 100 million different species on Earth, although nowhere near that many have been physically cataloged. Of these, the majority are Bacteria and Archaea.

**Another Example - Homo Sapiens**

Since there is no way to list all the different subdivisions of life on Earth here, we might as well focus on one specific animal: us, Homo sapiens. We are members of the Domain Eukarya, the Kingdom Animalia, the Phylum Chordata, the Class Mammalia, the Order Primates, the Family Hominidae, the Genus Homo, the Species Homo sapiens and finally the Subspecies Homo sapiens sapiens. This classification is able to demonstrate our exact biological position relative to life on Earth.

One important thing, a system like this tells us is that Homo, which is Latin for "human," is not actually our species, but our genus. This is an easy fact to forget since we are the only member of our genus not yet extinct. But anthropologically speaking there have been many humans including Homo habilis, Homo erectus and Homo neanderthalensis.

**Taxonomical classification is an evolutionary map**

Furthermore, the taxonomical classification system can be seen as a map of evolution on the planet. Plants, animals and bacteria can be traced back to common ancestors and newly discovered species can be classified relative to their ancestors, descendants and cousins. The Genus Homo, for instance, is a direct offshoot of the Tribe Hominini. (A tribe is a subcategory of the category of family, which here is Hominidae.) Another genus that falls under the Tribe Hominini is Pan, which houses the species Chimpanzee. This shows us that until relatively recently in the history of life, Homo sapiens and Chimpanzees were the same creature, and that Chimpanzees only split off just before Homo sapiens became fully human.

# Ecology

**Ecology is the scientific study of the relationship between the Earth and its life forms. The purpose of ecology is to understand the structures that occur in nature.**

Ecologists study the planet's ecosystems, the various communities of living things (biotic) and non-living structures (abiotic) that occur in localized areas throughout the world. The purpose of ecology is to understand the organizational structures that occur spontaneously in nature. Within an ecosystem there are different levels of organization which are broken down by relative size. Each ecosystem has communities of animals, and within each community exist numerous populations, or individual species groups.

## Ecosystems Ecology

**Ecosystems ecology studies areas that can be differentiated from neighboring areas by the types of rocks, soil and other non-living features, as well as the types of plants and animals adapted to live there.**

A desert ecosystem may boarder an arid grassland ecosystem, which in turn may boarder a forest ecosystem. The purpose of ecosystems ecology is to analyze the system of interactions the animals and plants in a particular area have with the non-living portions environment. It also focuses heavily on local evolution, studying what traits are favored within particular ecosystems and why.

**Ecosystems can be qualified.**

Many quantifiable factors go into making an ecosystem. Abiotic components are things such average sunlight, temperature, average rainfall and moisture levels, soil composition and other similar factors. Similarly, biotic components consist of the number and type of primary producers (generally plants), secondary producers (herbivores) and tertiary producers (carnivores and omnivores). All of this information can be quantified. For example, ecologists can calculate the amount of energy in a system by studying average amount of sunlight, the efficiency of photosynthesis in local plants, calories that exist in prey animals, nutrients absorbed by bacteria from breaking down dead predators and so on. Provided all of the factors have been accounted for, this sort of quantitative analysis of ecosystems can help ecologists determine factors such as the efficiency of the food web and the maximum supportable population. It can also help determine accurate ways to repair damaged ecosystems.

## Community Ecology

**Community ecology looks at similar regions to ecosystems ecology but focuses primarily on the biotic factors, ignoring the abiotic.**

In ecological terms a community describes the interactions of several species in a local area. Ecologists define these interactions between species in several ways: mutualism, interaction where both species benefit such as between bees and flowering plants; commensalism, interaction where one species benefits and the other neither notices nor minds; competition, interaction where both species are harmed; and predation or parasitism, interaction where one species is benefitted while the other is harmed such as predators attacking prey or herbivores eating plants.

**A local food web, is a graphical representation showing who eats what in nature.**

To ecologists, however, food webs are much more specific, showing the transfer of energy from organism to organism. Energy moves from lower trophic levels to higher ones. Trophic levels are the various positions that plants and animals occupy within the food web relative to other plants and animals that they want to eat or that want to eat them. Plants, for instance, would have a lower trophic level than grazing animals such as deer. Similarly, deer would have lower trophic levels than wolves.

Within communities species can be affected by changes either directly (such as when they are eaten by their main predator) or indirectly (such as when their main predator has its numbers diminished by a new and even bigger predator). There are also cascading effects on communities, such as when a dominant herbivorous species dies out and all its former prey (both plant and animal) increase drastically in number.

**Each organism occupies a trophic level (or position) in the food chain.**

A food chain represents a succession of organisms that eat another organism and are, in turn, eaten themselves. The number of steps an organism is from the start of the chain is a measure of its trophic level. The simplest, and first trophic level (level 1) are plants, then herbivores (level 2), and then carnivores (level 3).

## Population Ecology

**Population Ecology studies a single species and the primary factor is population size.**

Getting even more specific is population ecology, which focuses on only one species either within a community or across a large space. The primary characteristic of a population is its size. Population sizes can change due to an imbalance in the number of births and deaths as well as plants and animals emigrating to new areas.

Ecologists who study populations will generally model their growth rates to make predictions about the species. One method is the exponential growth model, which looks at current population trends and, assuming that they will remain constant, shows the increase or decrease in population over numerous generations. The other method is the logistic growth model, which slows reproduction when populations reach a certain density and increases it when they drop below a certain density to account for the increase in predators and decrease in the food supply that often follows massive population growth.

## Natural Selection and Adaptation

**Natural selection and adaptation are the fundamental teachings of evolution. Natural selection is the non-random gradual process that biological traits become more common or less common among a population.**

The theory of natural selection was made popular by Charles Darwin and was first introduced in his 1859 book; The Origin of Species.

As species and organisms evolve, some mutations and changes in the genomes occur as they interact with their environments. These changes and mutations can be passed from the organism to its offspring. In time, individual organisms or living beings with particular traits or genome variants may survive and produce offspring more successfully than individuals with different traits or genome variants. As this process goes on, the population slowly evolves as individuals with weak traits relative to their environment die out or are replaced by individuals with the right traits or mutations to survive. This is why the process of natural selection is also sometimes called the survival of fittest.

Over time as species and organisms continue to react to their environment and develop traits and genome variants to suit their environment they may become specialized to suit a particular environment niche, and new species may even be produced. Natural selection is thus an important pillar of evolution although it is not the only process that leads to evolution.

**Natural selection differs with artificial selection because the latter involves the purposeful selection of specific favorable traits by humans.**

With natural selection, the individual organism doesn't make the choice, but the changing environment determines which traits are necessary for survival and individual organisms that lack the required traits would die out.

**Not all variants and mutations affect the survival of the individual.**

For example, the difference in eye color among a population such as among humans is not necessarily a survival factor. However, a rabbit that develops the trait of running faster and passes it onto its offspring does have improved chances of escape and survival from predators than rabbits that do not. The same would be true for algae that successfully develop the trait or ability to extract more energy from sunlight, such algae would outgrow others without this trait.

**Adaptation**

**Adaptation is a process in which an organism evolves to be better able to live and survive in its habitat or environments.**
Adaptation is closely related to natural selection and it covers both the state of being adapted to the environment and the process that led to the adaptation. Adaptation is also a fundamental teaching of evolution as popularized by Charles Darwin.

**Organisms existing in their various environments face several challenges that they must adapt to to survive. An organism must develop observable phenotype traits in response to the conditions imposed on it by its environment for it to survive and thrive.**

The ability of an organism to adapt is thus closely linked to its fitness and survival. Adaptation is not exactly simple or fast. It may take a period of small steps for the entire process to be complete and for the organism to be fully adapted. During all the stages of adaptation and evolution, the organism has to be viable to be able to survive the process.

Adaptation is a process in which the phenotype of the organism changes to better suit the environment. There are many classical examples of adaptation. An animal that develops thick fur to survive the cold environment has adapted, just as the case of an animal that develops effective camouflage techniques to hide itself from predators.

**Adaptation can be behavioral, structural or physiological.**

Structural adaptation has to do with changes in physical features such as body covering, physical defense mechanism, size and shape and some internal restructuring.

Physiological adaptations allow the organism to do perform unique functions such as secreting slime, making venom or phototropism. Physiological adaptations include general functions such as temperature regulation, development and growth and ionic balance.

Behavioral adaptations include inherited behaviors and mannerisms as well as the ability to learn. Inherited behaviors are termed instinct and may include mating style, food search and vocalizations.

# Basic Concepts in Chemistry

## Atoms

**Atoms are some of the basic building blocks of matter. Each atom is an element—an identifiable substance that cannot be further broken down into other identifiable substances.**

There are just over 100 such elements, and each of them can combine with themselves and with other elements to create all the various molecules that exist in the universe. The poison gas chlorine and the explosive metal sodium, for instance, can combine at the atomic level to form sodium chloride, also known as salt.

For thousands of years atoms were thought to be the smallest thing possible. (The word "atom" comes from an ancient Greek word meaning "unbreakable.") However, experiments performed in the mid to late 19th century began to show the presence of small particles, electrons, in electric current. By the early 20th century, the electron was known to be a part of the atom that orbited a yet undefined atomic core. A few years later, in 1919, the proton was discovered and found to exist in the nuclei of all atoms.

**The protons and neutrons inside an atomic nucleus are not fundamental particles. That is, they can be divided into still smaller pieces.**

Protons and neutrons are known as hadrons, which is a class of particle made up of quarks. (Quarks are a fundamental particle.) There are two distinct types of hadrons, baryons and mesons, and both protons and neutrons are baryons, meaning they are both made up of a combination of three quarks. Besides being hadrons, protons and neutrons are also known as nucleons because of their place within the nucleus. Protons have a mass of around $1.6726 \times 10^{-27}$ kg and neutrons have a nearly identical mass of $1.6929 \times 10^{-27}$ kg. Both particles have a ½ spin.

**The number of protons inside an atomic nucleus determines what element the atom is.**

An element with only one proton, for instance, is hydrogen. An element with two is helium. One with three is lithium, and so on. No element (except for hydrogen) can exist with only protons in its nucleus. Atoms need neutrons to bond the protons together using the strong force. In general atoms (again except for hydrogen) have an equal number of protons and neutrons in their nuclei.

**Atoms with an uneven number of protons and neutrons are called isotopes.**

Isotopes have all the same chemical properties as their evenly balanced counterparts, but their nuclei are not usually as stable and are more willing to react with other elements. (Two deuterium atoms, hydrogen isotopes with one proton and one neutron in their nucleus rather than only one proton, will fuse much more readily than two regular hydrogen atoms.)

**Nearly all of an atoms' mass is within its nucleus. Outside that there is a lot of empty space occupied only by a few, tiny electrons.**

Electrons were once viewed as orbiting an atom like planets orbit the sun. We now know that this is wrong in several ways. For one, electrons do not really "orbit" in the sense we are used to. At the quantum level no particle is really a particle, but is actually both a particle and a wave simultaneously. Heisenberg's uncertainty principle looks at this odd truth about reality and says that you can never watch an electron orbit the nucleus as you would watch the Earth orbit the sun. Instead, you have to observe only one of the electron's physical characteristics at a time, either viewing it as a particle in a fixed position outside the nucleus or as a wave encircling the nucleus like a halo. Additionally, planets orbiting their stars can orbit at any distance they want. In fact, every object in our solar system has an elliptical orbit, meaning that they all move in more oval rather than circular shapes, getting closer and farther from the sun at various points. Electrons cannot do this under any circumstances.

**Atoms have what are known as electron shells, which are the levels that an electron is able to occupy.**

Electrons cannot exist in between these shells; instead they jump from one to the next instantaneously. Each electron shell can hold a different number of atoms. When a shell fills up, additional electrons fill the outer shells. The outermost shell of any atom is called the valence shell, and it is the electrons in this shell that interact with the electrons of other atoms. The important thing about the valence shell is that each electron shell has a specific number of electrons that it can hold, and it wants to hold that many.

**When atoms join, their connecting valence electrons take up two valence shell spots, one on each atom.**

This means that the fewer electrons an atom has in its valence shell, the likelier it is to interact with other atoms. Conversely, the more electrons it has, the less likely it is to interact.

**Electrons can also momentarily jump from one electron shell to the next if they are hit with a burst of energy from a photon.**

When photons hit atoms, the energy is briefly absorbed by the electrons, and this momentarily knocks them into higher "orbits." The particular "orbit" the electron is knocked into depends on the type of atom, and when the electron gives up its higher energy level it re-emits a photon at a slightly different wavelength than the one it absorbed, providing a characteristic signal of that atom and showing exactly what "orbit" the electron was knocked into.

**This is the phenomenon responsible for spectral lines in light and is the reason we can tell what elements make up stars and planets just by looking at them.**

Unlike protons and neutrons, electrons are a fundamental particle. They are known as leptons.

Electrons have a negative charge that is generally balanced out by the positive charge of their atom's protons.

**Charged atoms, which have either gained or lost an electron for various reasons, are called ions.**

Ions, like isotopes, have the same properties that the regular element does; they simply have different tendencies towards reacting with other atoms. Electrons have a mass of $9.1094 \times 10^{-31}$ kg and a $-\frac{1}{2}$ spin.

## Element

**The concept of chemical element is related to that of chemical substance. A chemical element is specifically a substance which has a single type of atom.**

A chemical element is characterized by the number of protons in the nuclei of its atoms. This number is known as the atomic number of the element. For example, all atoms with 6 protons in their nuclei are atoms of the chemical element carbon, and all atoms with 92 protons in their nuclei are atoms of the element uranium.

## Compound

**A compound is a substance with a particular ratio of atoms of particular chemical elements which determines its composition, and a particular organization which determines chemical properties.**

For example, water is a compound containing hydrogen and oxygen in the ratio of two to one, with the oxygen atom between the two hydrogen atoms, and an angle of 104.5° between them. Compounds are formed and interconverted by chemical reactions.

## Substance

**A chemical substance is a kind of matter with a definite composition and set of properties.**

Strictly speaking, a mixture of compounds, elements or compounds and elements is not a chemical substance, but it may be called a chemical. Most of the substances we encounter in our daily life are some kind of mixture; for example: air, alloys, biomass, etc.

**Nomenclature of substances is a critical part of the language of chemistry. Generally it refers to a system for naming chemical compounds.**

Earlier in the history of chemistry substances were given names by their discoverer, which often led to some confusion and difficulty. However, today the IUPAC system of chemical nomenclature allows chemists to specify by name specific compounds amongst the vast variety of possible chemicals.

The standard nomenclature of chemical substances is set by the International Union of Pure and Applied Chemistry (IUPAC). There are well-defined systems in place for naming chemical species. Organic compounds are named according to the organic nomenclature system. Inorganic compounds are named according to the inorganic nomenclature system. In addition the Chemical Abstracts Service has devised a method to index chemical substance. In this scheme each chemical substance is identifiable by a number known as CAS registry number.

# Molecule

**Molecules are two or more atoms join through a chemical bond to form chemicals.**

Molecules differ from atoms in that molecules can be further broken down into smaller pieces and into elements while atoms cannot. (This was actually the 18th century definition of an atom: a recognizable structure that could no longer be broken down into smaller bits.)

**Atoms are joined into molecules in two main ways: through covalent bonds and through ionic bonds.**

Covalent bonds are the primary type of chemical bond that forms molecules. They occur when atoms with only partially filled valence electron shells, an atom's outermost electron shell, come together to share electrons. Hydrogen atoms, for instance, each have only one electron, while their valence shell is capable of holding two. When two hydrogen atoms come together each share the other's electron, using it to occupy its valence shell's free space forming the H2 molecule: hydrogen gas.

**Not all covalent bond's are the same.**

Different atoms have different levels of positive charge coming from in their nuclei, and although, under normal circumstances, the negative charge of the atom's electrons balances that out (keeping the atom electrically neutral) the chemical bonding process has a way of exploiting this situation. If we look at the H2 molecule again, everyday experience tells us that it has a strong tendency to seek out and bond with oxygen (O) molecules forming H20, or water. There are two main reasons for this. The first comes from the regular old covalent bonds that are already holding H2 together. If bonded to another atom, hydrogen gains the ability to form a new valence shell that can hold six electrons. Since oxygen is the only molecule to naturally have six electrons in its valence shell, it is the most eager to bond with hydrogen. However, oxygen also has 8 protons in its nucleus compared to the total of 2 in the H2 molecule. This means that as the atoms come closer and prepare to bond, the electrons from both atoms are pulled closer to the oxygen molecule and farther from the hydrogen. An atom's proclivity to pull electrons towards itself is called its electronegativity, and this process creates polar covalent bonds. Due to this connection, polar covalent bonds are the strongest molecular bond, which is why molecules like water are so prevalent in our solar system and, likely, throughout the galaxy.

**One very interesting aspect of polar covalent bonds is the hydrogen bond.**

When a hydrogen atom bonds with another electronegative atom, the newly created molecule develops an intense polar attraction to all other electronegative atoms. This attraction works almost like a magnet with one end of the molecule exhibiting a positive charge (due to the effects of the polar covalent bonds pulling all the electrons towards one end of the molecule) and the other end exhibiting a negative charge. This phenomenon is responsible for, among other things, the way water molecules stick to each other so readily. This is why you can fill a glass of water to a millimeter or so above the rim before it spills.

**Hydrogen bonds are also responsible for how hydrophilic and hydrophobic molecules react to being mixed with water.**

Hydrophilic molecules are molecules like NaCl (salt) which exhibit their own strong charge for reasons we will discuss in a moment. The charged salt molecules mix eagerly with the charged water molecules due to the extra pull of the hydrogen bond. Conversely, hydrophobic molecules such as oil will not mix with water because they are neutrally charged and do not like charged molecules. This is the reason you have to shake up an oil based salad dressing each time you use it. Oil and the water never truly mix, and quickly separate.

**A very different type of bond between atoms is called the ionic bond.**

Ionic bonds only occur between ions, atoms that are either positively or negatively charged due to having an unequal number of protons and electrons. Ionic bonds always occur between metals and non-metals, such as the gas chlorine (Cl) and the alkaline metal sodium (Na). In their normal states, neither of these elements are ions, but when they approach, the sodium gives the chlorine one of its electrons forming Cl- and Na + ions, which subsequently become attracted. Since no electrons are actually lost, the molecule still technically has a neutral charge; it is only the atoms that are charged.

In ionic bonds it is always the metal which gives its electron to the non-metal. Additionally, in a diluted or liquid form, molecules that are created like this will always conduct electricity. This is why salt water can make such a good conductor.

## Ions and salts

**An ion is a charged species, an atom or a molecule, that has lost or gained one or more electrons.**

Positively charged cations (e.g. sodium cation Na+) and negatively charged anions (e.g. chloride Cl−) can form a crystalline lattice of neutral salts (e.g. sodium chloride NaCl). Examples of polyatomic ions that do not split up during acid-base reactions are hydroxide (OH−) and phosphate (PO43−).

Ions in the gaseous phase are often known as plasma.

## Acidity and basicity

**A substance can often be classified as an acid or a base. There are several different theories which explain acid-base behavior. The simplest is Arrhenius theory.**

The Arrhenius theory states than an acid is a substance that produces hydronium ions when it is dissolved in water, and a base is one that produces hydroxide ions when dissolved in water. According to Brønsted–Lowry acid-base theory, acids are substances that donate a positive hydrogen ion to another substance in a chemical reaction; by extension, a base is the substance which receives that hydrogen ion.

**A third common theory is Lewis acid-base theory, which is based on the formation of new chemical bonds.**

Lewis theory explains that an acid is a substance capable of accepting a pair of electrons from another substance during the process of bond formation, while a base is a substance which can provide a pair of electrons to form a new bond. According to concept as per Lewis, the crucial things being exchanged are charges. There are several other ways in which a substance may be classified as an acid or a base, as is evident in the history of this concept

**Acid strength is commonly measured by two methods. The most common is pH.**

One measurement, based on the Arrhenius definition of acidity, is pH, which is a measurement of the hydronium ion concentration in a solution, as expressed on a negative logarithmic scale. Thus, solutions that have a low pH have a high hydronium ion concentration, and can be said to be more acidic. The other measurement, based on the Brønsted–Lowry definition, is the acid dissociation constant ($K_a$), which measure the relative ability of a substance to act as an acid under the Brønsted–Lowry definition of an acid. That is, substances with a higher $K_a$ are more likely to donate hydrogen ions in chemical reactions than those with lower $K_a$ values.

# Phase

**In addition to the specific chemical properties that distinguish chemical classifications, chemicals can exist in several phases.**

For the most part, the chemical classifications are independent of these bulk phase classifications; however, some more exotic phases are incompatible with certain chemical properties. A phase is a set of states of a chemical system that have similar bulk structural properties, over a range of conditions, such as pressure or temperature.

Physical properties, such as density and refractive index tend to fall within values characteristic of the phase. The phase of matter is defined by the phase transition, which is when energy put into, or taken out of the system goes into rearranging the structure of the system, instead of changing the bulk conditions.

**Phase can be continuous.**

Sometimes the distinction between phases can be continuous instead of having a discrete boundary, here the matter is considered to be in a supercritical state. When three states meet based on the conditions, it is known as a triple point and since this is invariant, it is a convenient way to define a set of conditions.

The most familiar examples of phases are solids, liquids, and gases. Many substances exhibit multiple solid phases. For example, there are three phases of solid iron (alpha, gamma, and delta) that vary based on temperature and pressure. A principle difference between solid phases is the crystal structure, or arrangement, of the atoms. Another phase commonly encountered in the study of chemistry is the aqueous phase, which is the state of substances dissolved in aqueous solution (that is, in water).

Less familiar phases include plasmas, Bose-Einstein condensates and fermionic condensates and the paramagnetic and ferromagnetic phases of magnetic materials. While most familiar phases deal with three-dimensional systems, it is also possible to define analogs in two-dimensional systems, which has received attention for its relevance to systems in biology.

## Redox

**Redox is a concept related to the ability of atoms of various substances to lose or gain electrons.**

Substances that can oxidize other substances are said to be oxidative and are known as oxidizing agents, oxidants or oxidizers. An oxidant removes electrons from another substance. Similarly, substances that can reduce other substances are said to be reductive and are known as reducing agents, reductants, or reducers.

**A reductant transfers electrons to another substance, and is thus oxidized itself. And because it "donates" electrons it is also called an electron donor.**

Oxidation and reduction properly refer to a change in oxidation number—the actual transfer of electrons may never occur. Thus, oxidation is better defined as an increase in oxidation number, and reduction as a decrease in oxidation number.

## Bonding

**Electron atomic and molecular orbitals**

**Atoms sticking together in molecules or crystals are said to be bonded with one another.**

A chemical bond may be visualized as the multi-pole balance between the positive charges in the nuclei and the negative charges oscillating about them. More than simple attraction and repulsion, the energies and distributions characterize the availability of an electron to bond to another atom.

**A chemical bond can be a covalent bond, an ionic bond, a hydrogen bond or just because of Van der Waals force.**

> Each of these kinds of bond is ascribed to some potential. These potentials create the interactions which hold atoms together in molecules or crystals. In many simple compounds, Valence Bond Theory, the Valence Shell Electron Pair Repulsion model (VSEPR), and the concept of oxidation number can explain molecular structure and composition.

## Reaction

**During chemical reactions, bonds between atoms break and form, resulting in different substances with different properties.**

> In a blast furnace, iron oxide, a compound, reacts with carbon monoxide to form iron, a chemical elements, and carbon dioxide.

> When a chemical substance is transformed as a result of its interaction with another or energy, a chemical reaction is said to have occurred. Chemical reaction is therefore a concept related to the 'reaction' of a substance when it comes in close contact, as a mixture or a solution; exposure to some form of energy, or, both. It results in some energy exchange between the constituents of the reaction as well with the system environment which may be designed vessels which are often laboratory glassware.

**Chemical reactions can result in the formation or dissociation of molecules, that is, molecules breaking apart to form two or more smaller molecules, or rearrangement of atoms within or across molecules.**

> Chemical reactions usually involve the making or breaking of chemical bonds. Oxidation, reduction, dissociation, acid-base neutralization and molecular rearrangement are some of the commonly used kinds of chemical reactions.

> Chemical reactions are symbolically depicted through a chemical equation. While in a non-nuclear chemical reaction the number and kind of atoms on both sides of the equation are equal, for a nuclear reaction, this holds true only for the nuclear particles viz. protons and neutrons.

**The sequence of steps in which the reorganization of chemical bonds may be taking place in the course of a chemical reaction is called its mechanism.**

> A chemical reaction can be envisioned to take place in several steps, each of which may have a different speed. Many reaction intermediates with variable stability can thus be envisaged during a reaction. Reaction mechanisms are proposed to explain the kinetics and the relative product mix of a reaction. Many physical chemists specialize in exploring and proposing the mechanisms of various chemical reactions. Several empirical rules, like the Woodward-Hoffmann rules often come handy while proposing a mechanism for a chemical reaction.

## Equilibrium

**Although the concept of equilibrium is widely used across sciences, in the context of chemistry, it arises whenever several different states of the chemical composition are possible.**

For example, in a mixture of several chemical compounds that can react, or, when a substance can be present in more than one kind of phase.

A system of chemical substances at equilibrium even though having an unchanging composition is most often not static; molecules of the substances continue to react, thus creating a dynamic equilibrium. Thus the concept describes the state in which the parameters such as chemical composition remain unchanged over time. Chemicals present in biological systems are invariably not at equilibrium; but are far from equilibrium.

## The Periodic Table

**The periodic table contains the known chemical elements displayed in a special tabular arrangement based on their electron configurations, atomic numbers and recurring chemical properties.**

The first semblance of a periodic table was by Antoine Lavoisier in 1789. He published a list or table of the 33 chemical elements known as of that time. He grouped the elements into earths, non-metals, gases and metals. Several chemists in the next century looked for a better classification method resulting in the periodic table as we have it today.

### Structure of the Periodic Table

The standard periodic table today is an 18 column by 7 rows table containing the main chemical elements. Beneath that is a smaller 15 column by 2 rows table. The periodic table can be broken into 4 rectangular blocks: the P block is by the right, S block is left, D block is at the middle and the F block is underneath that. The elements in the blocks are based on which sub-shell the last electron resides.

The chemical elements on the table are arranged in order of increasing atomic number, which refers to the number of protons of the element. The periodic table can be used to study the chemical behavior of chemical elements, which makes it a very important tool widely used in chemistry.

The periodic table contains only chemical elements. Mixtures, compounds or small atomic particles of elements are not included. Each element on the table has a unique atomic number, which represents the number of protons contained in the element's nucleus.

A new period or row begins when an element has a new electron shell with a first electron. Columns or groups are based on the configuration of electrons of the atom. Elements that have an equal number of atoms in a specific sub-shell are listed under the same column. For example, selenium and oxygen both have 4 electrons in their outermost sub shell and so are listed under the P column. Elements with similar properties are listed in the same group although some elements in the same period can also share similar properties too. Since the elements grouped together have related properties, one can easily predict the property of an element if the properties of the surrounding elements are already known.

**Rows are Periods**

The rows of the periodic table are called periods. Elements on a row have the same number of electron shells or atomic orbitals. Elements on the first row have just one atomic orbital, elements on the second row have 2, and so it goes until the elements on the seventh row that have 7 electron shells or atomic orbitals.

**Columns are Groups**

Columns from up to down in the table are called groups. The columns in the D, P and S blocks are called groups. Elements within a group have an equal number of electrons in their outermost electron shell or orbital. The electrons on the outer shell are called valence electrons and there are the electrons that combine with other elements in a chemical reaction.

**The Periodic table contains natural and synthesized elements**

The elements up to californium are natural existing elements (94) while the rest were laboratory synthesized. Chemists are still working to produce elements beyond the present 118th element, ununoctium. 114 of the 118 elements on the table have been officially recognized by the International Union of Pure and Applied Chemistry (IUPAC). Elements listed on the table under 113, 115, 117 and 118 have been synthesized but are yet to officially recognized by the IUPAC and are only known by their systematic element names.

| Group → ↓ Period | 1 | 2 | 3 | 4 | 5 | 6 | 7 | 8 | 9 | 10 | 11 | 12 | 13 | 14 | 15 | 16 | 17 | 18 |
|---|---|---|---|---|---|---|---|---|---|---|---|---|---|---|---|---|---|---|
| 1 | 1 H | | | | | | | | | | | | | | | | | 2 He |
| 2 | 3 Li | 4 Be | | | | | | | | | | | 5 B | 6 C | 7 N | 8 O | 9 F | 10 Ne |
| 3 | 11 Na | 12 Mg | | | | | | | | | | | 13 Al | 14 Si | 15 P | 16 S | 17 Cl | 18 Ar |
| 4 | 19 K | 20 Ca | 21 Sc | 22 Ti | 23 V | 24 Cr | 25 Mn | 26 Fe | 27 Co | 28 Ni | 29 Cu | 30 Zn | 31 Ga | 32 Ge | 33 As | 34 Se | 35 Br | 36 Kr |
| 5 | 37 Rb | 38 Sr | 39 Y | 40 Zr | 41 Nb | 42 Mo | 43 Tc | 44 Ru | 45 Rh | 46 Pd | 47 Ag | 48 Cd | 49 In | 50 Sn | 51 Sb | 52 Te | 53 I | 54 Xe |
| 6 | 55 Cs | 56 Ba | | 72 Hf | 73 Ta | 74 W | 75 Re | 76 Os | 77 Ir | 78 Pt | 79 Au | 80 Hg | 81 Tl | 82 Pb | 83 Bi | 84 Po | 85 At | 86 Rn |
| 7 | 87 Fr | 88 Ra | | 104 Rf | 105 Db | 106 Sg | 107 Bh | 108 Hs | 109 Mt | 110 Ds | 111 Rg | 112 Cn | 113 Uut | 114 Fl | 115 Uup | 116 Lv | 117 Uus | 118 Uuo |

| | | 57 La | 58 Ce | 59 Pr | 60 Nd | 61 Pm | 62 Sm | 63 Eu | 64 Gd | 65 Tb | 66 Dy | 67 Ho | 68 Er | 69 Tm | 70 Yb | 71 Lu |
|---|---|---|---|---|---|---|---|---|---|---|---|---|---|---|---|---|
| Lanthanides | | | | | | | | | | | | | | | | |
| Actinides | | 89 Ac | 90 Th | 91 Pa | 92 U | 93 Np | 94 Pu | 95 Am | 96 Cm | 97 Bk | 98 Cf | 99 Es | 100 Fm | 101 Md | 102 No | 103 Lr |

## Basic Physics

### Kinetic and Mechanical Energy

**The kinetic energy of an object is the energy it possesses due to its motion.**

Kinetic energy is the work needed to accelerate a body of a given mass from rest to a stated velocity. Like all forms of energy, kinetic energy is measured in joules. Kinetic energy is imparted to an object when an energy source is tapped to accelerate it. It also happens when one object with kinetic energy slams into another object and kinetic energy from the first object is transferred to the second.

However it happens, imparting kinetic energy to an object causes it to accelerate. Movement, therefore, is nothing more than an indication of the amount of kinetic energy an object has. An object will hold onto its kinetic energy until it is able to transfer it to something else, which allows it to slow down again.

**While an object has the same level of kinetic energy, it will move at a consistent velocity forever. This is Newton's first law of motion.**

**The transfer of kinetic energy from one object to another can occur in many ways.**

The transfer of kinetic energy can be as simple and mundane as a baseball flying through the air—interacting with all the various molecules of oxygen, carbon dioxide, nitrogen and all the other gasses that make up our atmosphere, and transferring its kinetic energy to them—speeding them up and slowing itself down in the process. Or it can be as chaotic as a speeding truck losing control on an icy road and slamming into a wall.

**Different types of interactions between objects appear to be different but are in fact the same.**

The interaction between the baseball and the air and between the truck and the wall are only superficially different. One appears more chaotic than the other only because of the differences in mass between a baseball and a truck and the differences in "negative energy" possessed by free-floating air molecules compared to a solid wall. At its most basic, however, the same events are taking place in both examples. Molecules in the wall and the air scatter when the kinetic energy they receive causes them to move, and this produces heat and sound.

**Kinetic energy can be calculated with the formula KE = ½mv$^2$ where m is the mass of the object in kilograms, and v is its velocity in meters/second.**

**Kinetic energy increases by the square of an objects velocity.**

One important aspect of kinetic energy that makes it so potentially destructive is that the kinetic energy relative to not increase on pace with its velocity, but rather, relative to the square of its velocity. If you double an object's velocity, you will quadruple the kinetic energy it possesses (2²=4). If you quadruple the velocity, you increase the kinetic energy by sixteen times (4²=16). This leads to relatively small masses possessing very high kinetic energy levels when they are accelerated to only nominally high speeds. This is one reason why modern kinetic energy weapons (such as firearms) are able to cause large amounts of damage while being extremely compact.

## Mechanical Energy

**Mechanical energy is the ability of an object to do work.**

When discussing energy it is important to take a moment to understand mechanical energy and how it relates to the objects it interacts with. Mechanical energy is not a separate type of energy in the way that potential energy and kinetic energy differ.

**Mechanical energy is the potential energy available to an object added to all of the kinetic energy available to it, providing a total energy output.**

For instance, in our description of potential energy there is the example of a pole-vaulter hanging in mid-air with her pole bent at a near right angle to the ground. The bend in the pole-vaulter's pole contains elastic potential energy, which will help her clear the bar. However, that is not the only source of energy the pole-vaulter is restricted to. For anyone who has ever seen a track and field competition, you know that pole-vaulters take long, running starts before planting their poles in the ground. This imparts kinetic energy to the runners body, and it is that kinetic energy plus the pole's elastic potential energy that are added together in mid-air to impart the total mechanical energy that drives the pole-vaulter high into the air and over the bar.

## Potential Energy

**There are two main types of potential energy: gravitational potential energy and elastic potential energy.**

Potential energy is the potential an object has to act on other objects. As gravitational potential energy, the object is raised off the ground and is waiting for the force of gravity pulling at $9.8 m/s^2$, to grab hold of it and pull it towards the Earth.

This type of energy is very common in everyday life. It describes everything from a book falling off its shelf to a child tripping on a crack in the sidewalk. Because gravitational potential energy is so common, the equation describing it $PE_{grav}$ = mass * g * height should not be hard to figure out since it contains only easily observable features of matter: an object's mass, the force of gravity (g), and the object's height off the ground when it started falling.

Note that the height does not have to be measured from the ground. Any point can be chosen—such as a table top or even a point in mid-air—if you are only concerned with the energy an object would have if it fell from the point it was currently at to the point you have chosen.

**Gravitational Potential Energy Example**

If we take the example of a 1kg weight positioned at a height of 1 meter above the surface of Earth (where the gravity is $9.8m/s^2$—try this on Mars and you will get a different result), we end with the equation PEgrav = 1 * 9.8 * 1, which equals 9.8 joules of gravitational potential energy. A 1g weight positioned at the same height would be PEgrav = .001 * 9.8 * 1 or .0098J of potential energy, while a 1kg weight positioned a kilometer up would equal PEgrav = 1 * 9.8 * 1000 or 9800J of potential energy.

From this equation you may have picked up on the fact that the height an object is raised, is directly proportional to the amount of gravitational potential energy it has. Take a 1kg object and raise it to 5m, and you get 49J of potential energy. Double that to 10m, and you get 98J. Triple it to 15m and you will get 147J—three times the original 49J.

**Elastic Potential Energy**

**Elastic potential energy occurs when an object is stretched or compressed out of its normal "resting" shape. The quantity of energy that will be released when it finally returns to rest is the quantity of elastic potential energy it has while stretched or compressed.**

A common example of elastic potential energy is when an archer draws back the string of his bow. The farther back the bowstring is pulled, the more it will stretch. The more it stretches the more potential energy it will have waiting to send into the arrow.

**Elastic potential energy of an object can be determined using Hooke's law of elasticity. Hooke's law states that F = -kx where F is the force the material will exert as it returns to its resting state measured in Newtons, x is amount of displacement the material undergoes measured in meters, and k is the spring constant and is measured in Newtons/meter.**

To determine the potential energy of an elastic or springy material you use the equation $PE = 1/2\, kx^2$. According to this equation, an object such as a spring with a spring constant of 5N/m that is stretched 3 meters past its resting point would have a potential energy of 22.5J. That is, ½ * 5 * $3^2$ = 2.5 * 9 = 22.5J. Remember that elastic potential energy affects much more than just what you would consider elastic or springy material such as rubber bands, bungee cords and springs. There is elastic potential energy in a pole-vaulter's pole at the point where she is in the air and hanging onto a pole that is bent nearly sideways. In the next instant, her forward momentum will be boosted by the conversion of her pole's potential energy into kinetic energy, pushing her over the bar. Similarly, when a hockey player shoots the puck, he drags his stick along the ice as it moves forward, bending the shaft backwards slightly. This adds extra force to the puck as the stick snaps forward back into its normal resting position.

## Energy: Work and Power

**In the simplest terms, energy is the ability to do work.**

Energy allows objects and people to effect the physical world and displace (or move) other objects or people.

**Work in the physics sense is a very specific concept.**

Measured in joules, defined as being 1 Newton of force that displaces something by 1 meter. (J = Nm) As the mass of the object being displaced varies, the quantity of work in joules required to move it a meter will vary too.

**To determine the quantity of work being done, you can use the equation $W = F * d * \cos\Theta$.**

This defines work as the force applied, multiplied by the distance the object was displaced, multiplied by the cosine of $\Theta$ (Theta).

The force is measured in Newtons. Distance is measured in meters. The tricky part of this equation is determining the cosine of $\Theta$. $\Theta$ represents the difference in angle between the vector (or direction) the force is acting in and the vector the displacement is occurring. That means that there are really only three possible values for $\Theta$.

If the force is pushing or pulling in one direction, and the object being displaced is moving in that same direction, then there is no difference in angle between the vectors and $\Theta=0°$. This is the sort of force you get when a child pulls her sled across a snowy field. The direction the child is pulling and the direction the sled is traveling are the same. Since $\cos 0 = 1$ the quantity of work is determined simply by multiplying the force and the displacement.

Note that the angle of the vectors is determined by their relationship, and not to an ideal flat surface. That is, if the child is pulling her sled up a steep hill rather than across a field, the angle of $\Theta$ is still going to be 0° since the force she exerts on the sled and the sled itself are still traveling in the same direction.

The second possibility is when the force vector acts in the opposite direction of the object's displacement. This gives what is called "negative work" because the energy is working to hinder the object from moving rather than to help it. In this instance $\Theta=180°$ since the vector in which the force is acting and the vector in which the object is moving are opposite. This force is most commonly observed when dealing with friction.  It is the reason that hockey pucks and soccer balls will not travel forever; the force of friction exerted by the ice and by the grass is acting in the opposite direction.

The final difference in vectors is when the force being exerted on an object is at a right angle to its displacement.  Here, Θ=90°.  You can picture this as a waitress carrying a tray of drinks over to your table, and it provides for some odd conclusions.  Since the force we are talking about is the force the waitress is using to hold the tray vertically, but the displacement vector of the tray is horizontally across the room, we find that the force the waitress exerts no work at all.  It is not responsible for moving the tray horizontally towards your table.

This is represented mathematically with the fact that the cos90 = 0, meaning that the original equation W = F * d * cosΘ would be W = F * d * 0.  Without adding any additional information, it is obvious that work is going to equal zero joules.

**A different way to imagine this is to think of cargo in the back of a truck.**

It took work to load the cargo up onto the truck from the ground (the force vector and the displacement vector were both pointing in the same direction), but once the cargo was loaded, no additional work was required to keep it there.  The truck could drive from one end of the country to the other, but zero joules of work would be exerted keeping the cargo in place in the back of the truck.

**When you add a unit of time to your calculations of work, you get a new classification: power.**

Power is the rate at which work is done.  The equation that measures power, is power = work/time.  In this equation work is measured in joules, time is measured in seconds and power is measured in watts.
Since, as we noted above, one joule is the same as one Newton multiplied by one meter, this equation can also be written as power=(force*displacement)/time where force is measured in Newtons and displacement is measured in meters.  However, this opens further possibilities.  Since the math does not care if we first multiply force with displacement before dividing the whole thing by time, or we divide displacement by time, and then multiply the answer by force, we find the equation can also be written as power = force(displacement/time).

Given that displacement is measured in meters and the time in seconds, what we are really saying here is that power equals the amount of force applied to an object multiplied by that object's velocity (m/s).

**Thus we get two equations describing power: power = work/time and power=force*velocity.**

By definition, power has an inverse relationship with time; the less time that it takes for the work to be done, the more power is being applied. Power also has a direct relationship with force and velocity. Increase either the quantity of force being applied to an object, or the speed at which it is traveling, and you have increased the power.

## Defining Force and Newton's Three Laws

**In physics force is the term given to anything that has the power to act on an object, causing its displacement in one direction or another.**

to identify accurately, and therefore it took thousands of years to identify accurately and describe them. It was not until the 17th century that Isaac Newton described the basic physical forces and show how they acted on matter.

Force is measured using the unit Newton (N). One Newton can be defined with the formula $1N = 1kg(1m/s^2)$. In other words, if you accelerate a kilogram of matter by one meter per second per second, you have exerted one Newton of force on it.

**Newton developed three laws to explain the interactions of matter he observed. The first is often known as the "Law of Inertia."**

It states that an object at rest will stay at rest, and an object in motion will stay in motion, unless a force acts on it to change its state. This means that if you fire a spaceship out into the vacuum of space, and keep it clear from planets and stars that will apply force to it, the ship will keep going at the same speed forever.

This tendency to stay moving or stay at rest is known as inertia. Inertia is directly related to an object's mass; the more mass an object has, the more inertia it will have and the harder it will be to speed it up or slow it down. This is implied by the equation defining one Newton of force, but it is also obvious in everyday life. You have to exert more force to push a box of books across the floor than you would to push a box of clothes the same size. The box of books has more mass, so it has more inertia. Similarly, a baseball player can easily catch and stop a baseball thrown at over 100km/hr. If you were to ask that same player to stop a truck traveling at 100km/hr, you would get much less pleasant results.

**One important thing to remember about force is that it is a vector quantity, meaning that it points in a specific direction.**

Set a one kilogram object down on a table and you will have the force of gravity pulling it down at one Newton, and the force of all the atoms in the table pushing it up at one Newton. This is said to be a state of equilibrium, and it causes no change to the object's velocity. However, if the table had been poorly built and was only capable of pushing up at .75 Newtons, the object would pull through, snapping the table at its weakest points, and fall until it found something that was capable of applying the needed force to hold it up against gravity.

As such, an object can only be at rest if it has no forces acting on it, or if it has equal and opposite forces acting on it keeping it at equilibrium. If an unopposed force acts on an object, it will move.

**Newton's second law deals with what happens when you have the sort of unbalanced forces that we just described.**

It explains the movement of objects through the equation $F=ma$, where F is the force in Newtons, m is the object's mass in kilograms, and a is the object's acceleration in meters per second per second (m/s2).
Just like with Newton's first law, this equation shows that mass is very important when it comes to using a force to move objects. The larger the mass, the more force you will need to accelerate or decelerate it to the same velocity.

**Newton's third law states simply that for every action there is an equal and opposite reaction**.

This means that if I pound my hand down on my desk right now, my desk will also be hitting up at my hand with the exact same force. This may sound strange, but it is the reason that pounding your hand on your desk can damage your desk and hurt your hand at the same time. It is also the reason that baseball bats can snap while imparting force onto the ball, and why a moving car hitting stationary wall will damage both.

## Force: Friction

**Friction is the force that resists the motion of objects relative to other objects.**

When two surfaces move relative to each other, the force of friction is what slows them down. Friction applies to all matter, whether it is a book sliding down a slanting shelf, a soccer ball rolling on the ground or a baseball flying though the air. Friction is a constant opposing force that keeps things from traveling forever.

**Several laws describe how friction works.**

Amontons' first law of friction says that, "The force of friction is directly proportional to the applied load." His second law of friction says that, "The force of friction is independent of the apparent area of contact." Similarly, Coulomb's law of friction states that, "Kinetic friction is independent of the sliding velocity."

**The two main types of Friction are static friction and kinetic friction.**

Static friction is what you get when one stationary object is stacked on top of another stationary object, such as a book resting on a table. The static friction between the book and the table determines how much sticking power there is between them, and at what angle you would have to tilt the table before the force of gravity overpowers the force of friction and starts the book sliding.

To calculate the maximum amount of static friction possible before the book starts sliding, you use the formula $f_s = \mu_s F_n$ where $f_s$ is the total amount of static friction, $\mu_s$ (pronounced "mu") is the coefficient of static friction and $F_n$ is the "normal force," the force being exerted perpendicularly through the surface into the object resting on it, keeping the object from breaking through the surface.

**Another way to examine static friction is to calculate the angle the table will have to reach before the book will start sliding.**

This is also known as the angle of repose, and it can be calculated using the formula $\tan\theta = \mu_s$ where $\theta$ (pronounced "theta") is the angle of repose, and $\mu_s$ is the coefficient of static friction.

Aside from determining the angles that books will slide off tables, calculating static friction allows tire manufacturers to determine how "grippy" their treads are. If there were no friction, the wheel would not be a functional tool because it would not push itself against the road while moving. The higher the coefficient of friction between the tire and the road, the more grip the tire has.

**Kinetic friction is like the inverse of static friction.**

It is the force that causes moving objects to slow down. Kinetic friction applies to two surfaces moving relative to one another such as the bottom of a snowboard and the snowy ground. It can be calculated using the same basic formula used to calculate static friction: $f_k = \mu_k F_n$ with the only differences being the sub-k marks replacing the sub-s marks of the previous equation, signifying kinetic friction.

As kinetic friction slows an object, the object's kinetic energy is transformed into heat.

## Fundamental Forces: Electromagnetism

**Electromagnetism is one of the four fundamental forces. It is far more common than gravity, but only if you know where to look.**

Electromagnetism is responsible for nearly all interactions in which gravity plays no part. It is what holds negatively charged electrons in orbit around the positively charged protons in the nucleus of an atom. It is also the force that joins atoms to create molecules.

**It is also electromagnetism that is responsible for the fact that matter—which is made up of atoms and at the subatomic level is mostly empty space—feels solid.**

When you sit down in your chair, it is the electromagnetic attraction between the chair's atoms and between your body's atoms that keep you from falling through the chair and, conversely, that keep the chair from passing through you.

**Electromagnetic force acts through a field.**

This type of field can occur as a result of positively or negatively charged atoms (ions), atoms which have either more or fewer electrons than protons causing their overall charge to be unbalanced. Magnetic fields can also be created by applying electric current to conductive material (such as wire) with a conductive core (such as a nail).

**Electric current is nothing more than a steady flow of electrons, and by turning on the current you send electrons through the core.**

This aligns all the atoms in the metal so that they are parallel, and this creates a magnetic field. When you turn the electric current off, the electrons stop flowing, and the atoms, no longer forced by the current to line up, cease to be magnetic.

**All electromagnetic fields have a positive and a negative pole.**

Even the Earth's magnetic field, which is caused by the convective forces in the planet's core, sends electrons out of its negative pole (in the geographic North Pole) and reaccepts them at its positive pole (in the geographic South Pole in Antarctica). The Earth's magnetic field, like all magnetic fields, is able to effect charged particles.

**Magnetic fields move in one direction around a magnet.**

This direction is always the same relative to the flow of current from negative to positive poles, and it is easy to test the direction of the field using the "right hand rule." Close your fist and make a "thumbs up" sign with your right hand. The positive pole is represented by the tip of your thumb, the negative by the other end of your hand, and the direction of the magnetic field by where your closed fingers are. Thus, if you point your thumb at yourself, your magnet has current coming out its negative pole pointed towards you and looping back around to the positive pole pointed away from you, and the field is pointed counter-clockwise, which here is to your left.

**The effects of a magnetic field do not go on forever but follow the inverse square law.**

The farther you move from a magnetic field, the less its force will effect you. By moving x times away from a magnetic field, you feel 1/x2 times less magnetism.

**Closely related to the electromagnetic field is electromagnetic radiation.**

This radiation can take many forms, the most familiar are light, radio waves that carry radio and broadcast television, microwaves that cook our food, x-rays that can image the insides or our bodies, and gamma rays that come down from space and would have killed us all long ago if it were not for the Earth's magnetic field interacting with them.

**Electromagnetic radiation is created, according to James Clerk Maxwell, by the oscillations of electromagnetic fields, which create electromagnetic waves.**

The wave's frequency (or how energetic it is) determines what part of the electromagnetic spectrum it occupies—whether it is a gamma ray, a blue light or a radio signal. Electromagnetic radiation is the same thing as light, with what we are used to as visible light being a range of specific frequencies within the electromagnetic spectrum, so all electromagnetic radiation moves at the speed of light.

**At the quantum level, the electromagnetic force has a transfer particle moving between charged atoms, attracting and repelling them. The electromagnetic transfer particle is the photon.**

## Fundamental Forces: Gravity

**Gravity may be the most commonly, consciously experienced force.**

We can see its effects everyday when books fall off shelves, when stray baseballs arc downwards and crash through windows and when Australians time and again fail to fall off the bottom of the world and out into space. Gravity is also largely responsible for the structure of the universe. Without it, stars would not ignite and begin fusion reactions, planets would not condense out of dust and metal and most matter would have no attraction to other matter in any way. Without gravity, life would not exist.

**It may seem strange to learn that gravity is the weakest of all forces given that it holds the entire galaxy together.**

> Still, even with the gravitational mass of the entire planet pulling on an object such as a ball—causing it to sit motionless on the floor rather than float aimlessly off into space—a toddler could easily pick it up and run off with it, and there would be nothing the planet could do about it. Match that with the force an electromagnet exerts on metal; there is no comparison.

**The idea of gravity as a force was first formulated by Isaac Newton in the late 17th century.**

> Newton's ideas were further elaborated on in the early 20th century by Albert Einstein, who described gravity as the effect of mass warping the fabric of space-time. This process is often portrayed as a large ball creating a divot in a flat sheet of space-time. The divot curves space-time and can catch objects that would otherwise be traveling in straight lines and redirect or even capture them.

**On Earth gravity pulls objects towards the center of the planet at 9.8 m/s$^2$.**

> The squared rate of time shows that gravity is by its nature a force causing acceleration. Every second, the force of gravity increases the speed of an object by an additional 9.8 m/s, provided nothing able to resist the force gets in its way.

**In Einstein's view of the universe, gravity moved in waves, which traveled through space at the speed of light.**

> As a result, he demonstrated that the force of gravity would take time to reach the object it was acting on. If, for instance, the sun were to vanish suddenly from the solar system, it would take eight minutes for the Earth to go flying off into space—the same amount of time it would take for us to stop seeing the sun's light.

**Another way to view gravity is through a series of transfer particles that interact with matter and draw it closer together.**

> Transfer particles come into play in quantum mechanics, and they replace gravity waves as the method of spreading the force through the universe. (Actually, replace is not the right word, as quantum mechanics shows that particles and waves are really the same thing, simply looked at from different perspectives.) In quantum mechanics gravity's transfer particle is called a graviton, and it moves at the speed of light.

**The farther you move from a gravitational mass, the less its force will affect you.**

> The drop in the gravitational force is governed by what is known as the inverse square law, which says the attraction of any object drops relative to the square of the distance you move from it. If you are floating over the surface of the planet and then move x times away from it, you will feel $1/x^2$ times less gravity.

So if you move 10 times farther away from where you were, you will feel 1/100 the force gravity.

# Fundamental Forces: Strong and Weak Nuclear Forces

**The strong and weak nuclear forces are fundamental forces, but they were discovered much later than electromagnetism and gravity primarily because they only interact with matter at a subatomic level.**

**Strong nuclear force is the strongest of the four fundamental forces.**

> Strong nuclear force is 100 times stronger than the next strongest force, electromagnetism, and 1036 times the strength of the weakest force, gravity. That said, for the thousands of years people have studied physics, it never occurred to any one to even look for the strong force. That is because, despite the strong force's strength, it has such a limited range that it only interacts with matter across the distance of an atom's nucleus. In fact, its range is only about 10-15 meters, so small that the nuclei of the largest atoms—those filled with the highest number of protons and neutrons—are only just barely small enough for the strong force to keep working, making the nuclei of those atoms unstable.

**The strong force was not discovered until the 1930s when scientists discovered the neutron.**

> Until that time atomic nuclei were thought to consist of a collection of protons and electrons grouped together in such a way that kept them mutually attracted. With the discovery of the neutron, however, a new force was needed to hold positively charged protons together with uncharged neutrons.

**Strong Nuclear force interacts with Quarks.**

> The strong force actually does not interact directly with the protons and neutrons but with the fundamental particle that makes up protons and neutrons, quarks. Quarks come in three different color groupings: red, green and blue. (Quarks are not actually these colors; red, green and blue are just familiar names given to bits of matter that are utterly outside our experience as humans, to make them easier to comprehend.) The different colors of quarks combine to create protons and neutrons. Within each proton and neutron, the strong force holds the quarks together. That, in turn, bleeds out into the rest of the nucleus in a residual effect, holding the protons and neutrons together as well.

> Like the other fundamental forces, the strong force is mediated at the quantum level using a transfer particle known as a gluon. However, unlike the transfer particles for gravity and electromagnetism (gravitons and photons, respectively), gluons have mass. It is the gluon's mass that limits the area where it can spread the strong force to only within the nucleus.

**Weak nuclear force causes a type of radioactive decay.**

The other fundamental force operating inside the nucleus is the weak force. The weak force causes a specific type of radioactive decay called beta decay, so named because it causes the decaying atom to emit a beta particle, which can be either an electron or a positron (a form of anti-mater also known as an anti-electron), as a by product of changing into a different element.

Several things happen at once during beta decay, and we should look at each one individually. We saw while looking at the strong force that an atom's protons and neutrons are made up of smaller, fundamental particles called quarks, and it is the quarks that actually interact with the strong force. As it turns out, quarks are the only particle that interacts with all four fundamental forces, which means that inside the nucleus they are interacting with the weak force as well.

**Besides three different colors: red, blue and green, Quarks can be divided into six different flavors: up, down, charm, strange, top and bottom.**

Before we get to how the weak force interacts with quarks, there is something else you should know about them. We mentioned above that quarks come in three different colors: red, blue and green. However, they also can be divided into six different flavors: up, down, charm, strange, top and bottom. (This makes 18 different possible combinations of quark, each with a color and a flavor.) Of these flavors only up and down quarks are stable enough to form protons and neutrons.

**What the weak force does is switch up quarks to down quarks and down quarks to up quarks.**

This is actually the only thing that the weak force does, but it has several effects. First since quarks join to produce protons and neutrons (two up quarks and one down quark make a proton, while two down and one up quark make a neutron), the sudden change of one type of quark to another changes that combination. β– decay is beta decay where change of quarks causes a neutron to become a proton. This also causes the atom to emit an electron and a electron antineutrino. β + decay is the opposite, where a proton changes to a neutron and the atom emits a positron and an electron neutrino.

In both cases the decaying atom changes into a different kind of atom. In general, beta decay takes place in unstable isotopes (atoms that have a different number of protons and neutrons) and stabilizes the nucleus by equalizing the ratio of these particles. For instance, beta decay will turn the unstable plutonium 15 into far more stable strontium 16.

## Quantum Mechanics

**Quantum mechanics is the study of quanta, the most basic individual unit of any substance.**

Quantum mechanics began as a discipline within physics in 1900 when Max Planck determined that energy radiated as heat could not just radiate at any temperature, but that it could only rise and fall—and thus be emitted or absorbed—at certain, set levels. (Think of it as the difference between stairs and ramps. Stairs have set spaces where you can stand and set spaces where you cannot. Planck said that raising energy levels such as temperature was akin to climbing a set of stairs one step at a time.)

**Radiation that produces heat (and thus all electromagnetic radiation, including visible light) is made up of tiny little particles, which Planck named quanta from the Latin work "quantus," which means "how much."**

Planck developed an equation to describe this situation, $E = h\nu$ in which $\nu$ stood for the already well known frequencies of electromagnetic spectrum (and which in 1900 was thought of as only acting like a wave), h stood for a number called the Planck constant that equaled $6.63 \times 10^{-34}$ J s ("J s" is for Joule seconds), and E was the energy level for quanta of that frequency.

**In 1905 Albert Einstein used Planck's work to define the photon, which is one quantum of electromagnetic radiation.**

Photons are generally thought of as light, but only some energies of photons are visible. Photons can have any energy that corresponds to electromagnetic frequency, but instead of being a continuous wave, they are thought of as individual particles.

**Waves and particles are the same thing look at in different ways.**

The discovery of the particle aspect of a wave led to a realization that waves and particles were actually the same thing, looked at in different ways. This idea, called wave-particle duality, accounted for the centuries long debate between physicists over whether light was a wave or a particle, with each side producing compelling evidence to prove its thesis. As it turned out light—like everything in the universe—was both. This relationship was demonstrated by Louis de Broglie who developed the equation $p = h/\lambda$ showing that the Planck constant (h) divided by a particle's wavelength ($\lambda$, pronounced lambda) would equal its momentum (p). Since all particles are moving and have momentum, all particles have wavelengths.

**One of the most important aspects of wave-particle duality comes from studying atoms.**

The orbits of electrons around the atomic nuclei had at one time been thought to mimic the orbits of planets around the sun. Now, however, two important factors came into play to change that view. The first was the realization that electrons could only orbit at certain distances from the nucleus. When changing from one electron shell to the next, an electron would not take a gradual trajectory to its new home in the way a spaceship from Earth to Mars might. The electron would simply vanish from one shell and appear instantaneously at the next. In essence, electrons could also only display certain quanta of energy. They could have one energy level or another, but they could not exist in between.

**The second important thing that quantum mechanics showed physicists is that "orbit" does not describe electrons and is only symbolic.**

Since all particles are also waves, an electron could not simply be in one place at one time, but had to exist as across a range of areas as a frequency which described its momentum.

**The Heisenberg uncertainty principle states you can measure the position of an electron or the velocity, but not both at once.**

This seemingly nonsensical idea was explained mathematically though the Heisenberg uncertainty principle, which stated that it was possible to measure the exact position of a particle, and it was possible to measure the exact velocity of a particle, but you could not know both factors at once. In other words, measuring one would make it impossible to measure the other. This was an unavoidable fact of reality given de Broglie's equation; if you were moving you were spread out like a wave.

**No particles in the universe can be said to have definite positions in space.**

A strange side-effect of this was it meant that no particles in the universe could be said to have definite positions in space. Instead, everything had a likely position given its velocity. Matter could not be said to exist at certain points in space, it could merely have certain probabilities of existing at those points.

**Gravity is still a problem.**

The 21st century understanding of gravity comes from Einstein's work on Special and General Relativity. The various predictions made by Einstein's theories have been proven correct experimentally on numerous occasions, and evidently his ideas accurately explain reality. However, they do not mix with quantum mechanics.

**Physics has three zones which do not mix - relativity, quantum mechanics and Newtonian.**

It is possible to look at physics and think of there as being three distinct zones: relativity, which describes the very big and the very fast; quantum mechanics, which describes the very small; and Newtonian physics, which describes everything in between.

But Newtonian physics easily unifies with quantum theory since the chaos and weirdness at the individual wave-particle level smooths out as you add more and more particles together, which is what we see when we look at the macro world in which we live. (That is, when you look at an object in front of you, you see it existing in a definite point in space because so many particles make it up the probability that they will all end suddenly existing elsewhere—the way individual particles can—drops to nearly zero.) Additionally, three of the four fundamental forces, electromagnetism, the strong force and the weak force, can all be explained through quantum mechanics using their three transfer particles; photons, gluons and bosons. They have been unified. However, the use of a gravity transfer particle, the graviton, in models has been less successful at bringing the experimentally accurate predictions of relativity in line with the functioning of reality at the quantum level.

## States of Matter

**Matter on Earth can exist in three main states or phases: solid, liquid and gas. There is also a fourth phase, plasma, that occurs when matter is superheated.**

The primary difference between the different phases of matter is the behavior of molecules relative to the temperature the matter is exposed to. The lower the temperature, the closer together and more locked together the molecules are. The higher the temperature, the each other apart the molecules are, and the more they move relative to each other.

### Solid

**Solid matter exists in a state where its molecules are locked together in a rigid structure preventing them from moving and, as a result, solid matter is held together in a specific shape.**

There are two primary types of solids, each defined by the structures in which their molecules are held. When the molecules in solid matter maintain a uniform organization they form a polycrystalline structure. This is how molecules in metal, ice and salt are organized. Polycrystalline structures are generally a result of the molecules' ionic properties. Water molecules, for instance, are formed in such a way that there are distinct ends, one with two hydrogen atoms and one with a single oxygen atom. The structure of the atoms within a water molecule means these ends are charged, giving it what amount to poles and causing water molecules to join only in specific patterns. Under a microscope polycrystalline solids are generally described as resembling lattice work or a chain link fence, with the same pattern of molecules from one end to the other.

When molecule's electromagnetic properties do not incline them to form into particular structures, they glob together in whatever patterns they can. This produces amorphous solids, most notably foams, glass and many types of plastic. Amorphous solids have no regular pattern throughout their structure and, as a result, are poor conductors of heat and electricity.

## Liquid

**When solids are heated past a certain point, the electromagnetic bonds holding their molecules together loosen, and the molecules are able to move more freely.**

While the temperatures required for this to happen can vary widely, the particular physical qualities of a liquid are always the same. Liquids are considered to be fluids, which differ from solids primarily in their ability to take the shape of any container they are held in. This is the result of a less intense electromagnetic connection between the molecules than there is in solids; however, there is still enough, that liquids want to stay in the same place. This is why liquids still maintain a low density that is nearly identical to their densities in solid form, and why they will maintain a constant volume rather than just drift off the way gasses do.

Liquids also have a property known as viscosity, which describes their willingness to flow away from themselves. Liquids such as water and honey have a constant viscosity and are known as Newtonian fluids. Non-Newtonian fluids, such as a goopy mixture of water and cornstarch can change their viscosities.

## Gas

**The third state of matter that is commonly found on Earth is gas. Gasses are formed when matter is heated beyond its liquid state so that the electromagnetic bonds holding its molecules together are severed almost completely.**

Gasses are also considered fluids and like liquids have no definite shape. But unlike liquids they lack a definite volume and have an extremely low density compared to their solid forms.

Since gasses lack both a shape and a volume, they will expand to fill any container they are placed in. Left unbounded they will expand forever. Conversely, gasses are perfectly happy to compress together in an enclosed space. (However, the more molecules of a gas that are enclosed in a space, the higher the gas's pressure—the force exerted by the molecules on the container's surface—will be.) One interesting thing about this expansion and compression is that it will always be homogeneous, meaning that as a gas expands to fill a container, there will never be pockets of higher density of molecules with pockets of lower density of molecules. The molecules will expand to fill the container equally.

## Plasma

**Plasma is the next step up from a gas; it is when a gas's molecules become super heated to the point where the molecular bonds themselves break down and the atoms begin shedding their electrons.**

Although plasma is rarely found on Earth, it is the most common state of matter throughout the universe. (It is the primary state of matter in stars, for instance.) Plasma has some unique characteristics, not the least of which is that it is ionized, or electrically charged. In many ways plasma acts like a gas. It lacks any definite shape or volume, and it will homogeneously fill any container. However, it can also be manipulated by electromagnetic fields, which alters its shape or contains it. Plasma is a super-heated, magnetically charged gas.

## Speed, Acceleration and Force Problems

### Acceleration

Acceleration is the rate velocity changes over time. A car starts from a zero speed in a straight line at increasing speed, it is accelerating in the direction of travel. If the car changes direction at the same speed, this is by definition acceleration, though not described as such; passengers in linear acceleration experience a force pushing them straight back, and a sideways force if the direction changes.

The formula for acceleration = $A = (V_f - V_0)/t$ and is measured in meters per second$^2$.

Here is a typical question:

**A car starts from standing top and in 10 seconds is traveling 20/meters per second. What is the acceleration?**

 a. 0.5 m/sec$^2$
 b. 1.5 m/sec$^2$
 c. 1 m/sec$^2$
 d. 2 m/sec$^2$

The formula for acceleration = $A = (V_f - V_0)/t$
so A = (20 m/sec - 0 m/sec)/10 sec = 2 m/sec$^2$

### Speed

Speed is the rate of change of an objects position, or,
speed = (total distance traveled)/(total time taken).

Here is a typical question:

**A rocket travels 3000 meters in 5 seconds. How fast is it traveling?**

    a. 100 m/sec
    b. 200 m/sec
    c. 500 m/sec
    d. 600 m/sec

Speed = (total distance traveled)/(total time taken)
3000/5 = 600 meters per second.

## Force

An everyday definition of Force is the push or pull. The more scientific definition of Force is any influence that causes an object to change its movement or direction. Force is measured in Newtons, (usually N) named after Sir Isaac Newton, and his formulation of the Second Law of motion, F = ma, where F = force, m = mass and a = acceleration.

$1 N = 1 kg\, m/s^2$.

Therefore,

Force = Mass times Acceleration Measured in Newtons.
Acceleration is the change in speed over time.
Speed is the change in position over time.

Here is a typical question:
**How much force is needed to accelerate a car that weights 500 kg to 10 m/s$^2$?**

    a. 20,000 N
    b. 30,000 N
    c. 40,000 N
    d. 50,000 N

Force = Mass times Acceleration Measured in Newtons.
F = 500 X 10 = 50,000 N

## Momentum

Momentum is the sum of the mass of an object and its velocity. This means that momentum measures the force produced by an object's mass and velocity.

For example, a very heavy object moving fast has a large momentum—it takes a large and prolonged force to get a very heavy object up to this speed, and it takes a large and prolonged force to bring it to a stop afterwards. If the object were lighter, or moving more slowly, then it would have less momentum, and it would be easier (i.e. require less force) to bring it to a stop.

The formula for calculating momentum is = Momentum = mass x velocity
Or
P = MV
Where P = momentum, V = velocity and M = mass

Based on the above definition, clearly the momentum of a car and a bicycle both traveling at 20 m/s will not be the same, because although the velocity of the two objects are the same, their mass is different. The car would have greater momentum, due to its larger mass.
Note:

The SI unit for velocity = m/s
SI unit for Mass = kg
So therefore momentum = kg x m/s and the SI unit for momentum is kg x m/s

Momentum must always have a direction and so the final answer must reflect the direction of the momentum or velocity.

Here is a typical question:

**What is the momentum of a log weighing 700 kg that is rolling down a hill at 4.6 m/s?**

   a. 3220 kg x m/s down the hill
   b. 3320 kg x m/s
   c. 3320 down hill
   d. 3320 M

Answer: A

P = MV
P = 700 X 4.6
P = 3220 kg x m/s down the hill.

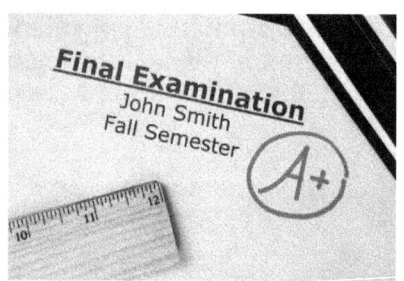

# PRACTICE TEST QUESTIONS SET 1

The questions below are not the same as you will find on the PAX RN - that would be too easy! And nobody knows what the questions will be and they change all the time. Below are general questions that cover the same subject areas as the PAX RN. So the format and exact wording of the questions may differ slightly, and change from year to year, if you can answer the questions below, you will have no problem with the PAX RN.

For the best results, take this Practice Test as if it were the real exam. Set aside time when you will not be disturbed, and a location that is quiet and free of distractions. Read the instructions carefully, read each question carefully, and answer to the best of your ability.

Use the bubble answer sheets provided. When you have completed the Practice Test, check your answer against the Answer Key and read the explanation provided.

Do not attempt more than one set of practice test questions in one day. After completing the first practice test, wait two or three days before attempting the second set of questions.

### Section I – Verbal Ability
**Questions:** 80 **Time:** 60 Minutes

### Section II – Mathematics
**Questions:** 50 **Time:** 60 Minutes

### Section III – Science
**Questions:** 75 **Time:** 60 minutes

# Answer Sheet – Verbal Ability

1. A B C D
2. A B C D
3. A B C D
4. A B C D
5. A B C D
6. A B C D
7. A B C D
8. A B C D
9. A B C D
10. A B C D
11. A B C D
12. A B C D
13. A B C D
14. A B C D
15. A B C D
16. A B C D
17. A B C D
18. A B C D
19. A B C D
20. A B C D
21. A B C D
22. A B C D
23. A B C D
24. A B C D
25. A B C D
26. A B C D
27. A B C D
28. A B C D
29. A B C D
30. A B C D
31. A B C D
32. A B C D
33. A B C D
34. A B C D
35. A B C D
36. A B C D
37. A B C D
38. A B C D
39. A B C D
40. A B C D
41. A B C D
42. A B C D
43. A B C D
44. A B C D
45. A B C D
46. A B C D
47. A B C D
48. A B C D
49. A B C D
50. A B C D
51. A B C D
52. A B C D
53. A B C D
54. A B C D
55. A B C D
56. A B C D
57. A B C D
58. A B C D
59. A B C D
60. A B C D
61. A B C D
62. A B C D
63. A B C D
64. A B C D
65. A B C D
66. A B C D
67. A B C D
68. A B C D
69. A B C D
70. A B C D
71. A B C D
72. A B C D
73. A B C D
74. A B C D
75. A B C D
76. A B C D
77. A B C D
78. A B C D
79. A B C D
80. A B C D

## Answer Sheet – Mathematics

1. A B C D
2. A B C D
3. A B C D
4. A B C D
5. A B C D
6. A B C D
7. A B C D
8. A B C D
9. A B C D
10. A B C D
11. A B C D
12. A B C D
13. A B C D
14. A B C D
15. A B C D
16. A B C D
17. A B C D

18. A B C D
19. A B C D
20. A B C D
21. A B C D
22. A B C D
23. A B C D
24. A B C D
25. A B C D
26. A B C D
27. A B C D
28. A B C D
29. A B C D
30. A B C D
31. A B C D
32. A B C D
33. A B C D
34. A B C D

35. A B C D
36. A B C D
37. A B C D
38. A B C D
39. A B C D
40. A B C D
41. A B C D
42. A B C D
43. A B C D
44. A B C D
45. A B C D
46. A B C D
47. A B C D
48. A B C D
49. A B C D
50. A B C D

# Answer Sheet – Science

1. A B C D
2. A B C D
3. A B C D
4. A B C D
5. A B C D
6. A B C D
7. A B C D
8. A B C D
9. A B C D
10. A B C D
11. A B C D
12. A B C D
13. A B C D
14. A B C D
15. A B C D
16. A B C D
17. A B C D
18. A B C D
19. A B C D
20. A B C D
21. A B C D
22. A B C D
23. A B C D
24. A B C D
25. A B C D
26. A B C D
27. A B C D
28. A B C D
29. A B C D
30. A B C D
31. A B C D
32. A B C D
33. A B C D
34. A B C D
35. A B C D
36. A B C D
37. A B C D
38. A B C D
39. A B C D
40. A B C D
41. A B C D
42. A B C D
43. A B C D
44. A B C D
45. A B C D
46. A B C D
47. A B C D
48. A B C D
49. A B C D
50. A B C D
51. A B C D
52. A B C D
53. A B C D
54. A B C D
55. A B C D
56. A B C D
57. A B C D
58. A B C D
59. A B C D
60. A B C D
61. A B C D
62. A B C D
63. A B C D
64. A B C D
65. A B C D
66. A B C D
67. A B C D
68. A B C D
69. A B C D
70. A B C D
71. A B C D
72. A B C D
73. A B C D
74. A B C D
75. A B C D

## Section I - Verbal Ability

**Directions:** The following questions are based on several reading passages. Each passage is followed by a series of questions. Read each passage carefully, and then answer the questions based on it. You may reread the passage as often as you wish. When you have finished answering the questions based on one passage, go right onto the next passage. Choose the best answer based on the information given and implied.

**Questions 1 – 4 refer to the following passage.**

**Passage 1 - The Life of Helen Keller**

Many people have heard of Helen Keller. She is famous because she was unable to see or hear, but learned to speak and read and went onto attend college and earn a degree. Her life is a very interesting story, one that she developed into an autobiography, which was then adapted into both a stage play and a movie. How did Helen Keller overcome her disabilities to become a famous woman? Read on to find out.
Helen Keller was not born blind and deaf. When she was a small baby, she had a very high fever for several days. As a result of her sudden illness, baby Helen lost her eyesight and her hearing. Because she was so young when she went deaf and blind, Helen Keller never had any recollection of being able to see or hear. Since she could not hear, she could not learn to talk. Since she could not see, it was difficult for her to move around. For the first six years of her life, her world was very still and dark.

Imagine what Helen's childhood was like. She could not hear her mother's voice. She could not see the beauty of her parent's farm. She could not recognize who was giving her a hug, or a bath or even where her bedroom was each night. Worse, she could not communicate with her parents in any way. She could not express her feelings or tell them the things she wanted. It must have been a very sad childhood.

When Helen was six years old, her parents hired her a teacher named Anne Sullivan. Anne was a young woman who was almost blind. However, she could hear and she could read Braille, so she was a perfect teacher for young Helen. At first, Anne had a very hard time teaching Helen anything. She described her first impression of Helen as a "wild thing, not a child." Helen did not like Anne at first either. She bit and hit Anne when Anne tried to teach her. However, the two of them eventually came to have a great deal of love and respect.

Anne taught Helen to hear by putting her hands on people's throats. She could feel the sounds people made. In time, Helen learned to feel what people said. Next, Anne taught Helen to read Braille, which is a way that books are written for the blind. Finally, Anne taught Helen to talk. Although Helen did learn to talk, it was hard for anyone but Anne to understand her.

As Helen grew older, she amazed more and more people with her story. She went to college and wrote books about her life. She gave talks to the public, with Anne at her side, translating her words. Today, both Anne Sullivan and Helen Keller are famous women who are respected for their lives' work.

**1. Helen Keller could not see and hear and so, what was her biggest problem in childhood?**

    a. Inability to communicate

    b. Inability to walk

    c. Inability to play

    d. Inability to eat

**2. Helen learned to hear by feeling the vibrations people made when they spoke. What were these vibrations were felt through?**

    a. Mouth

    b. Throat

    c. Ears

    d. Lips

**3. From the passage, we can infer that Anne Sullivan was a patient teacher. We can infer this because**

    a. Helen hit and bit her and Anne remained her teacher.

    b. Anne taught Helen to read only.

    c. Anne was hard of hearing too.

    d. Anne wanted to be a teacher.

**4. Helen Keller learned to speak but Anne translated her words when she spoke in public. The reason Helen needed a translator was because**

    a. Helen spoke another language.

    b. Helen's words were hard for people to understand.

    c. Helen spoke very quietly.

    d. Helen did not speak but only used sign language.

**Questions 5 – 7 refer to the following passage.**

**Passage 2 - Ways Characters Communicate in Theater**

Playwrights give their characters voices in a way that gives depth and added meaning to what happens on stage during their play. There are different types of speech in scripts that allow characters to talk with themselves, with other characters, and even with the audience.

It is very unique to theater that characters may talk "to themselves." When characters do this, the speech they give is called a soliloquy. Soliloquies are usually poetic, introspective, moving, and can tell audience members about the feelings, motivations, or suspicions of an individual character without that character having to reveal them to other characters on stage. "To be or not to be" is a famous soliloquy given by Hamlet as he considers difficult but important themes, such as life and death.

The most common type of communication in plays is when one character is speaking to another or a group of other characters. This is generally called dialogue, but can also be called monologue if one character speaks without being interrupted for a long time. It is not necessarily the most important type of communication, but it is the most common because the plot of the play cannot really progress without it.
Lastly, and most unique to theater (although it has been used somewhat in film) is when a character speaks directly to the audience. This is called an aside, and scripts usually specifically direct actors to do this. Asides are usually comical, an inside joke between the character and the audience, and very short. The actor will usually face the audience when delivering them, even if it's for a moment, so the audience can recognize this move as an aside.

All three of these types of communication are important to the art of theater, and have been perfected by famous playwrights like Shakespeare. Understanding these types of communication can help an audience member grasp what is artful about the script and action of a play.

**5. According to the passage, characters in plays communicate to**

    a. move the plot forward

    b. show the private thoughts and feelings of one character

    c. make the audience laugh

    d. add beauty and artistry to the play

**6. When Hamlet delivers "To be or not to be," he can be described as**

    a. solitary

    b. thoughtful

    c. dramatic

    d. hopeless

**7. The author uses parentheses to punctuate "although it has been used somewhat in film,"**

    a. to show that films are less important

    b. instead of using commas so that the sentence is not interrupted

    c. because parenthesis help separate details that are not as important

    d. to show that films are not as artistic

**Questions 8 – 11 refer to the following passage.**

**Passage 3 - Low Blood Sugar**

As the name suggest, low blood sugar is low sugar levels in the bloodstream. This can occur when you have not eaten properly and undertake strenuous activity, or, when you are very hungry. When Low blood sugar occurs regularly and is ongoing, it is a medical condition called hypoglycaemia. This condition can occur in diabetics and in healthy adults.

Causes of low blood sugar can include excessive alcohol consumption, metabolic problems, stomach surgery, pancreas, liver or kidneys problems, as well as a side-effect of some medications.

**Symptoms**

There are different symptoms depending on the severity of the case.

Mild hypoglycaemia can lead to feelings of nausea and hunger. The patient may also feel nervous, jittery and have fast heart beats. Sweaty skin, clammy and cold skin are likely symptoms.
Moderate hypoglycaemia can result in a short temper, confusion, nervousness, fear and blurring of vision. The patient may feel weak and unsteady.

Severe cases of hypoglycaemia can lead to seizures, coma, fainting spells, nightmares, headaches, excessive sweats and severe tiredness.

**Diagnosis of low blood sugar**

A doctor can diagnosis this medical condition by asking the patient questions and testing blood and urine samples. Home testing kits are available for patients to monitor blood sugar levels.  It is important to see a qualified doctor though.  A doctor can test to safely rule out other medical conditions that could affect blood sugar levels.

**Treatment**

Quick treatments include drinking or eating foods and drinks with high sugar contents. Good examples include soda, fruit juice, hard candy and raisins. Glucose energy tablets can also help. Doctors may also recommend medications and well as changes in diet and exercise routine to treat chronic low blood sugar.

**8. Based on the article, which of the following is true?**

a. Low blood sugar can happen to anyone.

b. Low blood sugar only happens to diabetics.

c. Low blood sugar can occur even.

d. None of the statements are true.

**9. Which of the following are the author's opinion?**

a. Quick treatments include drinking or eating foods and drinks with high sugar contents.

b. None of the statements are opinions.

c. This condition can occur in diabetics and in healthy adults.

d. There are different symptoms depending on the severity of the case

**10. What is the author's purpose?**

a. To inform

b. To persuade

c. To entertain

d. To analyse

**11. Which of the following is not a detail?**

a. A doctor can diagnosis this medical condition by asking the patient questions and testing.

b. A doctor will test blood and urine samples.

c. Glucose energy tablets can also help.

d. Home test kits monitor blood sugar levels.

d. None of the above.

**Questions 12 – 15 refer to the following passage.**

**How To Get A Good Nights Sleep**

Sleep is just as essential for healthy living as water, air and food. Sleep allows the body to rest and replenish depleted energy levels. Sometimes we may for various reasons have trouble sleeping which has a serious effect on our health. Those who have prolonged sleeping problems are facing a serious medical condition and should see a qualified doctor when possible for help. Here is simple guide that can help you sleep better at night.

Try to create a natural pattern of waking up and sleeping around the same time every day - avoid going to bed too early and sleeping past your usual wake up time. Going to bed and getting up at radically different times everyday confuses your body clock. Try to establish a natural rhythm as much as you can.

Exercises and a bit of physical activity can help you sleep better at night. If you are having problem sleeping, try to be as active as you can during the day. If you are tired from physical activity, falling asleep is a natural and easy process
for your body. If you remain inactive during the day, you will find it harder to sleep properly at night. Try walking, jogging, swimming or simple stretches close to your bed time.

Afternoon naps are great to refresh you during the day, but they may also keep you awake at night. If you feel sleepy during the day, get up, take a walk and get busy to keep from sleeping. Stretching is a good way to increase blood flow to the brain and keep you alert so that you don't sleep during the day. This will help you sleep better night.

> A warm bath or a glass of milk in the evening can help your body relax and prepare for sleep. A cold bath will wake you up and keep you up for several hours. Also avoid eating too late before bed.

**12. How would you describe this sentence?**

    a. A recommendation

    b. An opinion

    c. A fact

    d. A diagnosis

**13. Which of the following is an alternative title for this article?**

    a. Exercise and a good night's sleep

    b. Benefits of a good night's sleep

    c. Tips for a good night's sleep

    d. Lack of sleep is a serious medical condition

**14. Which of the following cannot be inferred from this article?**

    a. Biking is helpful for getting a good night's sleep

    b. Mental activity is helpful for getting a good night's sleep

    c. Eating bedtime snacks is not recommended

    d. Getting up at the same time is helpful for a good night's sleep

**15. What is a disadvantage of taking naps?**

   a. They may keep you awake.

   b. There are no disadvantages

   c. They may help you sleep better

   d. They may affect your diet

**Question 16 refers to the following Table of Contents.**

## Contents

   Science Self-assessment 81
   Answer Key 91
   Science Tutorials 96
   Scientific Method 96
   Biology 99
   Heredity: Genes and Mutation 104
   Classification 108
   Ecology 110
   Chemistry 112
   Energy: Kinetic and Mechanical 126
   Energy: Work and Power 130
   Force: Newton's Three Laws 132

**16. Consider the table of contents above. What page would you find information about natural selection and adaptation?**

   a. 81

   b. 90

   c. 110

   d. 132

**Questions 17 – 20 refer to the following passage.**

**Passage 5 - Pearl Harbor**

In 1941, the world was at war. The United States was trying to stay out of the conflict. In Europe, the countries of Germany and Italy had formed an alliance to expand their land and territory. Germany had already taken over Poland, Denmark, and parts of France. They were heading next toward England and due to all the fighting in Europe, there were battles taking place as far south as North Africa, where the German and Italian armies were fighting the British.

This got even worse when the Asian nation of Japan formed an alliance with Germany and Italy. Together, the three countries called themselves, the AXIS. Now, the war was in the Pacific as well as in Europe and Northern Africa. Many Americans thought that perhaps now was the time for the United States to join with its ally, Great Britain and stop the Axis from taking over more regions of the world.

In 1941, Franklin Roosevelt was President of the United States. His fear at the time was that Japan would try to take over many countries in Asia. He did not want to see that happen, so he moved some of the United States warships that had been stationed in San Diego, to the military base at Pearl Harbor, in Honolulu, Hawaii.

Japan quietly plotted their attack. They waited until the early hours of the morning on Sunday, December 7, 1941. Then, 350 Japanese war plans began to drop bombs on the U.S. ships at Pearl Harbor. The first bombs fell at 7:48 a.m. and only 90 minutes later, the attack was over. Pearl Harbor was decimated. 8 battleships were damaged. Eleven ships were sunk and 300 U.S. planes were destroyed. Most devasting was the loss of life 2,400 U.S. military members was killed in the attack and 1, 282 were injured.

President Roosevelt addressed the country via the radio and said "Today is a day that will live in infamy." He asked Congress to declare war on Japan. War was declared on Japan on December 8th and on Germany and Italy on December 11th. The United States had entered World War Two.

**17. After reading the passage, what can we infer infamy means?**

  a. Famous

  b. Remembered in a good way

  c. Remembered in a bad way

  d. Easily forgotten

**18. What three countries formed the Axis?**

  a. Italy, England, Germany

  b. United States, England, Italy

  c. Germany, Japan, Italy

  d. Germany, Japan, United States

**19. What do you think was President Roosevelt's reason for moving warships to Pearl Harbor?**

  a. He feared Japan would bomb San Diego

  b. He knew Japan was going to attack Pearl Harbor

  c. He was planning to attack Japan

  d. He wanted to try to protect Asian countries from Japanese takeover

**20. Why do you think Japan chose a Sunday morning at 7:48 am for their attack?**

    a. They knew the military slept late

    b. There is a law against bombing countries on a Sunday

    c. They wanted the attack to catch people by surprise

    d. That was the only free time they had to attack.

**Questions 21 - 24 refer to the following recipe.**

**If You Have Allergies, You're Not Alone**

People who experience allergies might joke that their immune systems have let them down or are seriously lacking. Truthfully though, people who experience allergic reactions or allergy symptoms during certain times of the year have heightened immune systems that are, "better" than those of people who have perfectly healthy but less militant immune systems.

Still, when a person has an allergic reaction, they are having an adverse reaction to a substance that is considered normal to most people. Mild allergic reactions usually have symptoms like itching, runny nose, red eyes, or bumps or discoloration of the skin. More serious allergic reactions, such as those to animal and insect poisons or certain foods, may result in the closing of the throat, swelling of the eyes, low blood pressure, inability to breath, and can even be fatal.

Different treatments help different allergies, and depend on the nature and severity of the allergy. It is recommended to patients with severe allergies to take extra precautions, such as carrying an EpiPen, which treats anaphylactic shock and may prevent death, always in order for the remedy to be readily available and more effective. When an allergy is not so severe, treatments may be used just relieve a person of uncomfortable symptoms. Over the counter allergy medicines treat milder symptoms, and can be bought at any grocery store and used in moderation to help people with allergies live normally.

There are many tests available to assess whether a person has allergies or what they may be allergic to, and advances in these tests and the medicine used to treat patients continues to improve. Despite this fact, allergies still affect many people throughout the year or even every day. Medicines used to treat allergies have side-effects, and it is difficult to bring the body into balance with the use of medicine. Regardless, many of those who live with allergies are grateful for what is available and find it useful in maintaining their lifestyles.

**21. According to this passage, which group does the word "militant" belong in**

    a. sickly, ailing, faint

    b. strength, power, vigor

    c. active, fighting, warring

    d. worn, tired, breaking down

**22. The author says that "medicines used to treat allergies have side-effects of their own" to**

    a. point out that doctors aren't very good at diagnosing and treating allergies

    b. argue that because of the large number of people with allergies, a cure will never be found

    c. explain that allergy medicines aren't cures, and some compromise must be made

    d. argue that more wholesome remedies should be researched and medicines banned

**23. It can be inferred that _____ recommend that some people with allergies carry medicine with them.**

    a. the author

    b. doctors

    c. the makers of EpiPen

    d. people with allergies

**24. The author has written this passage to**

    a. inform readers on symptoms of allergies so people with allergies can get help

    b. persuade readers to be proud of having allergies

    c. inform readers on different remedies so people with allergies receive the right help

    d. describe different types of allergies, their symptoms, and their remedies

**Questions 25 – 26 refer to the following email.**

SUBJECT: MEDICAL STAFF CHANGES

To all staff:

This email is to advise you of a paper on recommended medical staff changes has been posted to the Human Resources website.

The contents are of primary interest to medical staff, other staff may be interested in reading it, particularly those in medical support roles.

The paper deals with several major issues:

    1. Improving our ability to attract top quality staff to the hospital, and retain our existing staff. These changes will make our position and departmental names internationally recognizable and comparable with North American and North Asian departments and positions.

2. Improving our ability to attract top quality staff by introducing greater flexibility in the departmental structure.

3. General comments on issues to be further discussed relative to research staff.

The changes outlined in this paper are significant. I encourage you to read the document and send to me any comments you may have, so that it can be enhanced and improved.

Gordon Simms
Administrator,
Seven Oaks Regional Hospital

**25. Are all hospital staff required to read the document posted to the Human Resources website?**

    a. Yes all staff are required to read the document.

    b. No, reading the document is optional.

    c. Only medical staff are required to read the document.

    d. none of the above are correct.

**26. Have the changes to medical staff been made?**

    a. Yes, the changes have been made.

    b. No, the changes are only being discussed.

    c. Some of the changes have been made.

    d. None of the choices are correct.

**Questions 27 – 30 refer to the following passage.**

**When a Poet Longs to Mourn, He Writes an Elegy**

Poems are an expressive, especially emotional, form of writing. They have been in literature virtually from the time civilizations invented the written word. Poets often portrayed as moody, secluded, and even troubled, but this is because poets are introspective and feel deeply about the current events and cultural norms they are surrounded with. Poets often produce the most telling literature, giving insight into the society and mind-set they come from. This can be done in many forms.

The oldest types of poems often include many stanzas, which may or may not rhyme, and are more about telling a story than experimenting with language or words. The most common types of ancient poetry are epics, which are usually extremely long stories that follow a hero through his journey, or ellegies, which are often solemn in tone and used to mourn or lament something or someone. The Mesopotamians are often said to have invented the written word, and their literature is among the oldest in the world, including the epic poem titled "Epic of Gilgamesh." Similar in style and length to "Gilgamesh" is "Beowulf," an ellegy written in Old English and set in Scandinavia. These poems are often used by professors as the earliest examples of literature.

The importance of poetry was revived in the Renaissance. At this time, Europeans discovered the style and beauty of ancient Greek arts, and poetry was among those. Shakespeare is the most well-known poet of the time, and he used poetry not only to write poems but also to write plays for the theater. The most popular forms of poetry during the Renaissance included villanelles, (a nineteen-line poetic form) sonnets, as well as the epic. Poets during this time focused on style and form, and developed very specific rules and outlines for how an exceptional poem should be written.

As often happens in the arts, modern poets have rejected the constricting rules of Renaissance poets, and free form poems are much more popular. Some modern poems would read just like stories if they weren't arranged into lines and stanzas. It is difficult to tell which poems and poets will be the most important, because works of art often become more famous in hindsight, after the poet has died and society can look at itself without being in the moment. Modern poetry continues to develop, and will no doubt continue to change as values, thought, and writing continue to change.

Poems can be among the most enlightening and uplifting texts for a person to read if they are looking to connect with the past, connect with other people, or try to gain an understanding of what is happening in their time.

**27. In summary, the author has written this passage**

    a. as a foreword that will introduce a poem in a book or magazine

    b. because she loves poetry and wants more people to like it

    c. to give a brief history of poems

    d. to convince students to write poems

**28. The author organizes the paragraphs mainly by**

    a. moving chronologically, explaining which types of poetry were common in that time

    b. talking about new types of poems each paragraph and explaining them a little

    c. focusing on one poet or group of people and the poems they wrote

    d. explaining older types of poetry so she can talk about modern poetry

**29. The author's claim that poetry has been around "virtually from the time civilizations invented the written word" is supported by the detail that**

    a. Beowulf is written in Old English, which is not really in use any longer

    b. epic poems told stories about heroes

    c. the Renaissance poets tried to copy Greek poets

    d. the Mesopotamians are credited with both inventing the word and writing "Epic of Gilgamesh"

**30. According to the passage, the word "telling" means**

    a. Speaking

    b. Significant

    c. Soothing

    d. Wordy

## Verbal Ability Part II – Vocabulary

**31. Choose a verb that means fearless or invulnerable to intimidation and fear.**

    a. Feeble

    b. Strongest

    c. Dauntless

    d. Super

**32. Choose a word that means the same as the underlined word.**

**I see the differences when they are placed side-by-side and <u>juxtaposed.</u>**

    a. Compared

    b. Eliminated

    c. Overturned

    d. Exonerated

**33. Choose the best definition of regicide.**

    a. v. To endow or furnish with requisite ability, character, knowledge and skill

    b. n. Killing of a king

    c. adj. Disposed to seize by violence or by unlawful or greedy methods

    d. v. To refresh after labor

**34. Choose the best definition of pernicious.**

a. Deadly
b. Infectious
c. Common
d. Rare

**35. Fill in the blank.**

**After she received her influenza vaccination, Nan thought that she was _____ to the common cold.**

a. Immune
b. Susceptible
c. Vulnerable
d. At risk

**36. Choose a word that means the same as the underlined word.**

**She performed the gymnastics and stretches so well! I have never seen anyone so <u>nimble</u>.**

a. Awkward
b. Agile
c. Quick
d. Taut

**37. Choose a word that means the same as the underlined word.**

**Are there any more <u>queries</u>? We have already had so many questions today.**

a. Questions
b. Commands
c. Obfuscations
d. Paradoxes

**38. Choose a verb that means to remove a leader or high official from position.**

a. Sack
b. Suspend
c. Depose
d. Dropped

**39. Choose the best definition of pedestrian.**

a. Rare
b. Often
c. Walking or Running
d. Commonplace

**40. Choose the best definition of petulant.**

a. Patient
b. Childish
c. Impatient
d. Mature

**41. Fill in the blank.**

**Paul's rose bushes were being destroyed by Japanese beetles, so he invested in a good _____.**

a. Fungicide
b. Fertilizer
c. Sprinkler
d. Pesticide

**42. Choose the best definition of salient.**

a. adj. To make light by fermentation, as dough
b. adj. Not stringent or energetic
c. adj. Negligible
d. adj. Worthy of note or relevant

**43. Choose the best definition of sedentary.**

   a. n. A morbid condition, due to obstructed excretion of bile or characterized by yellowing of the skin

   b. adj. Not moving or sitting at a place

   c. v. To wander from place to place

   d. n. Perplexity

**44. Fill in the blank.**

**The last time that the crops failed, the entire nation experienced months of _____.**

   a. Famine

   b. Harvest

   c. Plenitude

   d. Disease

**45. Choose the best definition of stint.**

   a. Thrifty

   b. Annoyed

   c. Dislike

   d. Insult

**46. Choose the best definition of precipitate.**

   a. To rain

   b. To throw down

   c. To throw up

   d. To snow

**47. Choose the verb that means to build up or strengthen relative to morals or religion.**

   a. Sanctify

   b. Amplify

   c. Edify

   d. Wry

**48. Choose the noun that means exit or way out.**

   a. Door-jamb

   b. Egress

   c. Regress

   d. Furtherance

**49. Choose the best definition of the underlined word.**

**The tide was in this morning but now it is starting to recede.**

   a. Go out

   b. Flow

   c. Swell

   d. Come in

**50. Choose the word that means private, personal.**

   a. Confidential

   b. Hysteric

   c. Simplistic

   d. Promissory

**51. Choose the best definition of the underlined word.**

**I don't think that will make it any better - it is just going to aggravate the situation.**

   a. Worsen

   b. Precipitate

   c. Elongate

   d. None of the above

**52. Choose the best definition of the underlined word.**

**I didn't think this was her first appearance, but it is her debut.**

a. Exit
b. Introduction
c. Curtain Call
d. Resignation

**53. Fill in the blank.**

**Because of a pituitary dysfunction, Karl lacked the necessary _____ to grow as tall as his father.**

a. Glands
b. Hormones
c. Vitamins
d. Testosterone

**54. Choose the best definition of importune.**

a. To find an opportunity
b. To ask all the time
c. Cannot find an opportunity
d. None of the above

**55. Choose the best definition of sedulous.**

a. n. The support on or against which a lever rests
b. adj. Constant steady pursuit
c. v. To oppose with an equal force
d. n. The branch of medical science that relates to improving health

**56. Choose the best definition of tincture.**

a. n. Alcoholic drink with plant extract used for medicine
b. n. An artificial trance-sleep
c. n. A special medicinal drink made by mixing water with plant extracts
d. adj. The point of puncture

**57. Choose the noun that means serious criminal offence that is punishable by death or imprisonment above a year**

a. Trespass
b. Hampers
c. Felony
d. Obligatory

**58. Choose the best meaning of the underlined word.**

**His library is enormous. I didn't realize he was such a bibliophile.**

a. Book lover
b. Audiophile
c. Bibliophobe
d. Audiophobe

**59. Fill in the blank.**

**When Mr. Davis returned from southern Asia, he told us about the _____ that sometimes swept the area, bringing torrential rain.**

a. Monsoons
b. Hurricanes
c. Blizzards
d. Floods

**60. Choose the best definition of volatile.**

   a. Not explosive
   b. Catches fire easily
   c. Does not catch fire
   d. Explosive

# Section II – Math

**1. What is 1/3 of 3/4?**

   a. 1/4
   b. 1/3
   c. 2/3
   d. 3/4

**2. What fraction of $1500 is $75?**

   a. 1/14
   b. 3/5
   c. 7/10
   d. 1/20

**3. Add $-3x^2 + 2x + 6$ and $-x^2 - x - 1$.**

   a. $-2x^2 + x + 5$
   b. $-4x^2 + x + 5$
   c. $-2x^2 + 3x + 5$
   d. $-4x^2 + 3x + 5$

**4. 3.14 + 2.73 + 23.7 =**

   a. 28.57
   b. 30.57
   c. 29.56
   d. 29.57

**5. Find the mean of these set of numbers – 200,000, 10,020, 30,000, 15,000 1080**

   a. 1080
   b. 15,000
   c. 256,100
   d. 51,220

**6. What is 0.27 + 0.33 expressed as a fraction?**

   a. 3/6
   b. 4/7
   c. 3/5
   d. 2/7

**7. What is (3.13 + 7.87) X 5?**

   a. 65
   b. 50
   c. 45
   d. 55

**8. Express $3^4$ in standard form**

   a. 81
   b. 27
   c. 12
   d. 9

**9. What is 2/4 X 3/4 reduced to lowest terms?**

   a. 6/12
   b. 3/8
   c. 6/16
   d. 3/4

10. If a = 2 and y = 5, solve xy³ - x³

   a. 240
   b. 258
   c. 248
   d. 242

11. Three tenths of 90 equals:

   a. 18
   b. 45
   c. 27
   d. 36

12. Find the mean of these set of numbers – 1, 2, 3, 4, 5, 6, 7, 8, 9, 10

   a. 55
   b. 5.5
   c. 11
   d. 10

13. .4% of 36 equals

   a. 1.44
   b. .144
   c. 14.4
   d. 144

14. 5x + 3 = 7x -1. Find x

   a. 1/3
   b. 1/2
   c. 1
   d. 2

15. Find 2 numbers that sum to 21 and the sum of the squares is 261.

   a. 14 and 7
   b. 15 and 6
   c. 16 and 5
   d. 17 and 4

16. 5x + 2(x + 7) = 14x – 7. Find x

   a. 1
   b. 2
   c. 3
   d. 4

17. 5(z + 1) = 3(z + 2) + 11. Find z

   a. 2
   b. 4
   c. 6
   d. 12

18. What are the prime factors of 81?

   a. 3 x 3 x 9
   b. 3 x 27
   c. 3 x 3 x 3 x 3
   d. All of the above

19. The price of a book went up from $20 to $25. What percent did the price increase?

   a. 5%
   b. 10%
   c. 20%
   d. 25%

**20.** After taking several practice tests, Brian improved the results of his GRE test by 30%. If the first time he took the test, Brian answered 150 questions correctly, how many questions did he answer correctly on the second test?

    a. 105
    b. 120
    c. 180
    d. 195

**21.** Simplify $4^3 + 2^4$

    a. 45
    b. 108
    c. 80
    d. 48

**22.** A square lawn has an area of 62,500 square meters. How much will it cost to build a fence around it at a rate of $5.5 per meter?

    a. $4000
    b. $4500
    c. $5000
    d. $5500

**23.** A javelin is thrown into a field at 18m/s. if the Javelin weighs 1.5kg, what is the momentum?

    a. 1.2 kg x m/s into the field
    b. 12 kg x m/s into the field
    c. 27 kg x m/s into the field
    d. 2.7 kg x m/s into the field

**24.** Convert 204 to scientific notation

    a. $2.04 \times 10^{-2}$
    b. $0.204 \times 10^2$
    c. $2.04 \times 10^3$
    d. $2.04 \times 10^2$

**25.** There are 15 yellow and 35 orange balls in a basket. How many yellow balls must be added to make the yellow balls 65%?

    a. 35
    b. 50
    c. 65
    d. 70

**26.** If 144 students need to go on a trip and the buses each carry 36 students, how many buses are needed?

    a. 2
    b. 3
    c. 4
    d. 4.5

**27.** Using the factoring method, solve the quadratic equation: $x^2 + 4x + 4 = 0$

    a. 0 and 1
    b. 1 and 2
    c. 2
    d. -2

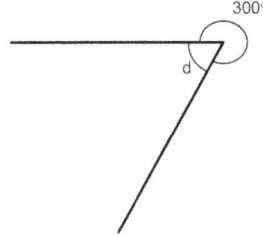

**28. What is the measurement of the indicated angle?**

   a. 45°
   b. 90°
   c. 60°
   d. 50°

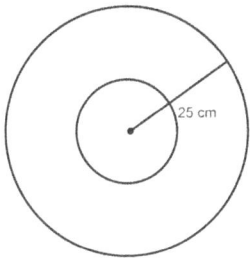

Note: figure not drawn to scale

**29. What is the distance travelled by the wheel above, when it makes 175 revolutions?**

   a. 87.5 π m
   b. 875 π m
   c. 8.75 π m
   d. 8750 π m

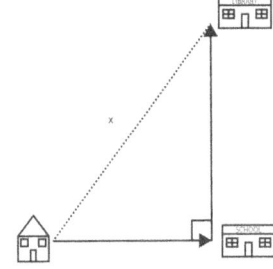

Note: figure not drawn to scale

**30. Every day starting from his home Peter travels due east 3 kilometers to the school. After school he travels due north 4 kilometers to the library. What is the distance between Peter's home and the library?**

   a. 15 km
   b. 10 km
   c. 5 km
   d. 12 ½ km

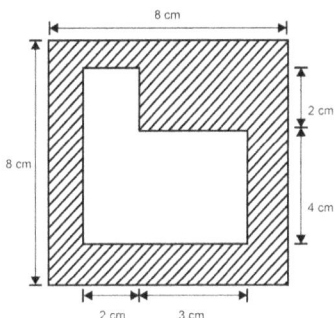

Note: figure not drawn to scale

**31. What is the area of the shaded region in the figure above?**

   a. 64 cm²
   b. 44 cm²
   c. 60 cm²
   d. 40 cm²

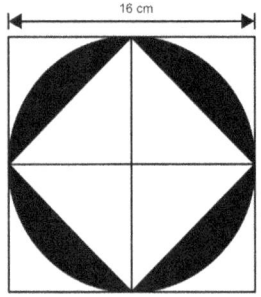

Note: figure not drawn to scale

**32. A tile factory makes custom tiles, shown above, from two types of stone. If a customer requires 200 tiles, how much black stone will be required?**

    a. 256 m²

    b. 2560 m²

    c. 2.56 m²

    d. 25.6 m²

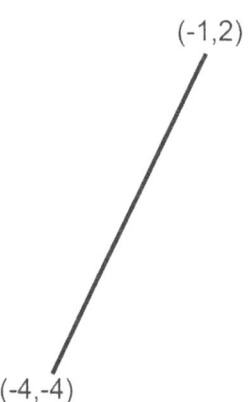

**33. What is the slope of the line above?**

    a. 1

    b. 2

    c. 3

    d. -2

**34. A caterer is hired for a wedding and needs to calculate how much wine is needed. The couple for her weddings always gets two liters of wine. Each guest receives 0.20 liters. If y is the amount of wine needed in total liters, and if x is the number of wedding guests, which equation below should be used calculate the number of liters the caterer will need?**

    a. y = 0.20x + 2

    b. y = 2x + 0.20

    c. y = 2.20x

    d. x = 0.20y + 2

**35. If we know it takes 12 men to operate four machines, how many are required for 20 machines?**

    a. 6

    b. 20

    c. 60

    d. 9

**36. Brad has agreed to buy everyone a Coke. Each drink costs $1.89, and there are 5 friends. Estimate Brad's cost.**

    a. $7

    b. $8

    c. $10

    d. $12

**37. An object that weighs 500g is rolling along the road at 3.5m/s, what is the momentum of the object?**

    a. 124.9 kg x m/s along road

    b. 17. 50 kg x m/s along road

    c. 1750 kg x m/s along road

    d. 1.75 kg x m/s along road

**38. Solve √121**

  a. 11
  b. 12
  c. 21
  d. None of the above

**39. What are the prime factors of 25?**

  a. 4 x 5.5
  b. 5 x 5 x 5
  c. 1 x 25
  d. 5 x 5

**40. Convert 0.00002011 to scientific notation**

  a. $2.011 \times 10^{-4}$
  b. $2.011 \times 10^{5}$
  c. $2.011 \times 10^{-6}$
  d. $2.011 \times 10^{-5}$

**41. Express the ratio of 7:25 as a percentage.**

  a. 20%
  b. 22%
  c. 25%
  d. 28%

**42.**

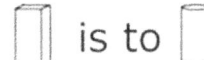
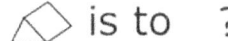

  a. ⬤   b. ▭
  c. ⬠   d. ⌭

**43.**

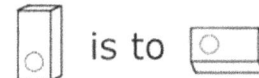
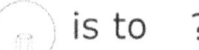

  a. ○   b. ◳
  c. ◉   d. ◉

**44.**

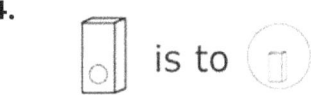
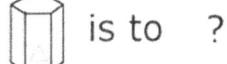

  a. △   b. ◰
  c. △   d. ▯

**45. Simplify the following expression:**

$3x^3 + 2x^2 + 5x - 7 + 4x^2 - 5x + 2 - 3x^3$

  a. $6x^2 - 9$
  b. $6x^2 - 5$
  c. $6x^2 - 10x - 5$
  d. $6x^2 + 10x - 9$

**46. A building is 15 m long and 20 m wide and 10 m high. What is the volume of the building?**

  a. 45 m³
  b. 3,000 m³
  c. 1500 m³
  d. 300 m³

**47. What is 465,890 less 456,890?**

   a. 9,000
   b. 7000
   c. 8970
   d. 8500

**48. Solve 3/4 + 2/4 + 1.2**

   a. 1 1/7
   b. 2 3/4
   c. 2 9/20
   d. 3 1/4

**49. A map uses a scale of 1:2,000. How much distance on the ground is 5.2 inches on the map if the scale is in inches?**

   a. 100,400
   b. 10, 500
   c. 10,440
   d. 10,400

**50. A bag contains 38 black balls and 42 white balls. What is the ratio of black balls to white?**

   a. 9:11
   b. 1:3
   c. 19:21
   d. 11:9

## Section III – Science

**1. A motorcycle is travelling at 90 mph accelerates to pass a truck. Five seconds later, it is going 120 mph. Calculate the motorcycles' acceleration**

   a. 6 mph/second$^2$
   b. 10 mph/second$^2$
   c. 15 mph/second$^2$
   d. 20 mph/second$^2$

**2. Which of the following disciplines have a close relationship with cell biology?**

   a. Genetics
   b. Genealogy
   c. Paleontology
   d. Archaeology

**3. A solution with a pH value of greater than 7 is**

   a. Base
   b. Acid
   c. Neutral
   d. None of the above

## 4. Ohm's law states

a. The voltage across a resistor is not equal to the product of the resistance and the current flowing through it.

b. The voltage across a resistor is equal to the product of the resistance and the current flowing through it.

c. The voltage across a resistor is greater than the product of the resistance.

d. The voltage across a resistor is equal to the current flowing through it.

## 5. Which statement below regarding Eukaryotic and prokaryotic cells is correct?

a. Both are organelles

b. Eukaryotic are not organelles

c. Both have DNA

d. Both have single membrane compartments

## 6. Electricity is a general term encompassing a variety of phenomena resulting from the presence and flow of electric charge. Which of the following statements about electricity is/are true?

a. Electrically charged matter is influenced by, and produces, electromagnetic fields.

b. Electric current is a movement or flow of electrically charged particles.

c. Electric potential is a fundamental interaction between the magnetic field and the presence and motion of an electric charge.

d. An influence produced by an electric charge on other charges in its vicinity is an electric field.

## 7. Which of these is not a process involved in cellular biology?

a. Active transport

b. Adhesion

c. Subversion

d. Cell signaling

## 8. When we say that important traits for scientific classification are homologous, "homologous" means

a. Being shared among two or more animals with the same parent.

b. Being coincidentally shared by two totally different creatures.

c. Being inherited by the organisms' common ancestors.

d. Mutating beyond all reasonable expectations.

**9. The manner in which instructions for building proteins, the basic structural molecules of living material are written in the DNA, is**

    a. Genotypic assignment

    b. Chromosome pattern

    c. Genetic code

    d. Genetic fingerprinting

**10. A _____ is a unit of inherited material, encoded by a strand of DNA and transcribed by RNA.**

    a. Allele

    b. Phenotype

    c. Gene

    d. Genotype

**11. A runner can sprint 6 meters per second. How far will she travel in 2 minutes?**

    a. 600 meters

    b. 720 meters

    c. 760 meters

    d. 800 meters

**12. Which of these is not an area studied in cell biology?**

    a. Cells physiological properties

    b. Cell structure

    c. Cell life cycle

    d. Cellular scientists' biographies

**13. Why is detection of pathogens complicated?**

    a. They evolve so quickly

    b. They die so quickly

    c. They are invisible

    d. They multiply so quickly

**14. Calculate the molarity of a sugar solution if 4 liters of the solution contains 8 moles of sugar?**

   a. 0.5 M

   b. 8 M

   c. 2 M

   d. 80 M

**15. Which of the following is/are not included in Ohm's Law?**

   a. Ohm's Law defines the relationships between (P) power, (E) voltage, (I) current, and (R) resistance.

   b. One ohm is the resistance value through which one volt will maintain a current of one ampere.

   c. Using Ohm's Law, voltage is determined using V = IR, with I equaling current and R equaling resistance.

   d. An ohm ($\Omega$) is a unit of electrical voltage.

**16. How many elements are represented on the modern periodic table?**

   a. 122 elements

   b. 99 elements

   c. 102 elements

   d. 118 elements

**17. Which, if any, of the following statements are false?**

   a. A mutation is a permanent change in the DNA sequence of a gene.

   b. Mutations in a gene's DNA sequence can alter the amino acid sequence of the protein encoded by the gene.

   c. Mutations in DNA sequences usually occur spontaneously.

   d. Mutations in DNA sequences can caused by exposure to environmental agents such as sunshine.

**18. Three cars are travelling down an even road at a velocity of 110 m/s, calculate the car with the highest momentum if they are all moving at the same speed, but the first car weighs 2500 kg, second car weighs 2650 kg and third car weighs 2009 kg?**

   a. First car

   b. Second car

   d. Third car

   d. All have same momentum

**19. Starting with the weakest, arrange the fundamental forces of nature in order of strength.**

    a. Gravity, Weak Nuclear Force, Electromagnetic Force, Strong Nuclear Force

    b. Weak Nuclear Force, Gravity, Electromagnetic Force, Strong Nuclear Force

    c. Strong Nuclear Force, Weak Nuclear Force, Electromagnetic Force, Gravity

    d. Gravity, Strong Nuclear Force, Weak Nuclear Force, Electromagnetic Force

**20. What are electrons?**

    a. Subatomic particles that carry a negative charge

    b. Subatomic particles that carry a positive charge

    c. Subatomic particles that carry both a negative and positive charge

    d. None of the above

**21. Cell culture is defined as**

    a. The technique for growing cells independent of a living organism within the confines of a laboratory.

    b. The process of killing cells through use of lasers.

    c. The method of creating cellular communities.

    d. A method for localizing proteins in tissue slices.

**22. _____, which refers to the repeatability of measurement, does not require knowledge of the correct or true value.**

    a. Precision

    b. Value

    c. Certainty

    d. Accuracy

**23. How much force is needed to accelerate a car weighing 2,000 kg, at a rate of 3 m/s$^2$?**

    a. 6000 N

    b. 10,000 N

    c. 4000 N

    d. 8000 N

**24. Describe the periodic table.**

a. The periodic table is a tabular display of the chemical compounds organized by their atomic numbers, electron configurations, and recurring chemical properties.

b. The periodic table is a tabular display of the chemical elements, organized by their atomic numbers, electron configurations, and recurring chemical properties.

c. The periodic table is a tabular display of the chemical subatomic particles, organized by their atomic numbers, electron configurations, and recurring chemical properties.

d. None of the above.

**25. The scientific discipline that studies the physiological aspects, structures, life cycles and division of cells is called _____.**

a. Physiology

b. Cell science

c. Biochemistry

d. Cell biology

**26. What is the minimum amount of energy required to remove an electron from an atom or ion in the gas phase?**

a. Ionization energy

b. Valence energy

c. Atomic energy

d. Ionic energy

**27. In a redox reaction, the number of electrons lost is**

a. Less than the number of electrons gained

b. More than the number of electrons gained

c. Equal to the number of electrons gained

d. None of the above

**28. In terms of the scientific method, the term _____ refers to the act of noticing or perceiving something and/or recording a fact or occurrence.**

a. Observation

b. Diligence

c. Perception

d. Control

**29. The _____ Theory defines acids and bases in terms of the electron-pair concept; according to its definition, an acid is an electron-pair acceptor, and a base is an electron-pair donor.**

   a. Arrhenius

   b. Lewis

   c. Clark

   d. Brønstead-Lowry

**30. What is the molarity of a solution containing 5 moles of solute in 250 milliliters of solution?**

   a. 20 M

   b. 15 M

   c. 0.104 M

   d. 1.25 M

**31. The property of a conductor that restricts its internal flow of electrons is:**

   a. Friction

   b. Power

   c. Current

   d. Resistance

**32. Describe bacteria.**

   a. Prokaryotic microorganisms that are usually just a few micrometers long.

   b. A single-celled organism.

   c. A virus.

   d. Three or more molecules clumped together.

**33. What is the difference, of any, between kinetic energy and potential energy?**

   a. Kinetic energy is the energy of a body that results from heat while potential energy is the energy possessed by an object that is chilled.

   b. Kinetic energy is the energy of a body that results from motion while potential energy is the energy possessed by an object by virtue of its position or state, e.g., as in a compressed spring.

   c. There is no difference between kinetic and potential energy; all energy is the same.

   d. Potential energy is the energy of a body that results from motion while kinetic energy is the energy possessed by an object by virtue of its position or state, e.g., as in a compressed spring.

**34. A rocket releases a satellite into orbit around Earth. The satellite travels at 2000 m/s in 25 seconds. What is the acceleration?**

    a. 60 m/sec²

    b. 80 m/sec²

    c. 100 m/sec²

    d. 120 m/sec²

**35. Name the four states in which matter exists.**

    a. Concrete, liquid, gas, and plasma

    b. Solid, fluid, gas, and plasma

    c. Solid, liquid, vapor, and plasma

    d. Solid, liquid, gas, and plasma

**36. Which one of the following best describes the function of a cell membrane?**

    a. It controls the substances entering and leaving the cell.

    b. It keeps the cell in shape.

    c. It controls the substances entering the cell.

    d. It supports the cell structures

**37. Describe electric current.**

    a. Electric current is the flow of voltage

    b. Electric current is the movement of negative ions.

    c. Electric current is the flow of electric charge through a medium.

    d. None of the above

**38. Which of the following is not a typical shape for a bacterium?**

    a. Rod

    b. Spiral

    c. Sphere

    d. Cube

**39. What is usually the result when acid reacts with most of the metals?**

    a. Carbon dioxide

    b. Oxygen gas

    c. Nitrogen gas

    d. Hydrogen gas

**40. Which of these is not a rank within the area of classification or taxonomy?**

a. Species

b. Family

c. Genus

d. Relative position

**41. Which of the following statements about the periodic table of the elements is true?**

a. On the periodic table, the elements are arranged according to their atomic mass.

b. The way in which the elements are arranged allows for predictions to made about their behavior.

c. The vertical columns of the table are called rows.

d. The horizontal rows of the table are called groups.

**42. The scientific term _____ refers to a practical test designed with the intention that its results be relevant to a particular theory or set of theories.**

a. Procedure

b. Variable

c. Hypothesis

d. Experiment

**43. Substances that deactivate catalysts are called**

a. Inhibitors

b. Catalytic poisons

c. Positive catalysts

d. None of the above

**44. What is the force per unit area exerted against a surface by the weight of air above that surface in the Earth's atmosphere?**

a. Gravitational force

b. Atmospheric pressure

c. Barometric density

d. Aneroid pressure

**45. Describe kinetic energy.**

   a. Kinetic energy is the energy an object possesses due to its mass.
   b. Kinetic energy is the energy an object possesses due to its motion.
   c. Kinetic energy is the energy an object possesses due to its chemical properties.
   d. Kinetic energy is the stored energy an object possesses.

**46. Another term for biological classification is:**

   a. Darwinian classification
   b. Animal classification
   c. Molecular classification
   d. Scientific classification

**47. When do oxidation and reduction reactions occur?**

   a. One after the other
   b. In separate reactions
   c. On the product side of the reaction
   d. Simultaneously

**48. What type of gene is not expressed as a trait unless inherited by both parents?**

   a. Principal gene
   b. Latent gene
   c. Recessive gene
   d. Dominant gene

**49. A _____ _____ is an approximation or simulation of a real system that omits all but the most essential variables of the system.**

   a. Scientific method
   b. Independent variable
   c. Control group
   d. Scientific model

**50. How many moles of Na are needed to make 4.5 liters of a 1.5 M Na solution?**

   a. 3 mol
   b. 0.33 M
   c. 0.33 mol
   d. 3 M

**51. Neutrons are necessary within an atomic nucleus because**

a. They bind with protons via nuclear force

b. They bind with nuclei via nuclear force

c. They bind with protons via electromagnetic force

d. They bind with nuclei via electromagnetic force

**52. How do atoms of different elements combine to form chemical mixtures?**

a. Atoms of different elements combine in simple whole-number ratios to form chemical compounds.

b. Atoms of different components combine in simple fractional ratios to form chemical compounds.

c. Atoms of the same element combine in simple whole-number ratios to form chemical compounds.

d. Atoms of different elements combine in simple whole-number ratios to form chemical mixtures.

**53. Which of the following statements is false?**

a. Most enzymes are proteins

b. Enzymes are catalysts

c. Most enzymes are inorganic

d. Enzymes are large biological molecules

**54. _____ are compounds that contain hydrogen, can dissolve in water to release hydrogen ions into solution, and, in an aqueous solution, can conduct electricity.**

a. Caustics

b. Bases

c. Acids

d. Salts

**55. Find the momentum of a round stone weighing 12.05 kg rolling down a hill at 8 m/s.**

a. 95 kg m/sec down the hill.

b. 96.4 kg m/sec down the hill.

c. 100 kg m/sec down the hill.

d. 90 kg m/sec down the hill.

**56. Which of the following statements about non-metals are false?**

a. A non-metal is a substance that conducts heat and electricity poorly.
b. Most known chemical elements are non-metals.
c. A non-metal is brittle or waxy or gaseous.
d. None of the statements are false.

**57. What is the name of the discipline that studies bacteria?**

a. Bacteriography
b. Bacteriology
c. Bacteriepathy
d. Bacterioscopy

**58. What are the basic structural units of nucleic acids (DNA or RNA) whose sequence determines individual hereditary characteristics?**

a. Gene
b. Nucleotide
c. Phosphate
d. Nitrogen base

**59. Which of these statements about light energy is/are true?**

a. Light consists of electromagnetic waves in the visible range.
b. The fundamental particle or quantum of light is a photon.
c. A and B are true.
d. None of the statements are true.

**60. List the classifications of organisms in order of size.**

a. Genus, Kingdom, Phylum/division, Class, Order, and Family Species
b. Order, Kingdom, Phylum/division, Genus, Class, and Family Species
c. Genus, Kingdom, Phylum/division, Class, Order, and Family Species
d. Kingdom ,Genus, Phylum/division, Class, Order, and Family Species

**61. Explain chemical bonds.**

a. Chemical bonds are attractions between atoms that form chemical substances containing two or more atoms.

b. Chemical bonds are attractions between protons that form chemical elements containing two or more atoms.

c. Chemical bonds are two or more atoms that form chemical substances.

d. None of the above

**62. The number of protons in the nucleus of an atom is the**

a. Atomic mass.

b. Atomic weight.

c. Atomic number.

d. None of the above.

**63. The molarity of an aqueous solution of CaCl is defined as the**

a. moles of CaCl per milliliter of solution

b. grams of CaCl per liter of water

c. grams of CaCl per milliliter of solution

d. moles of CaCl per liter of solution

**64. An electron is:**

a. A tiny particle with a negative charge.

b. A tiny particle with a positive charge.

c. A tiny particle with a negative charge that orbits a nucleus.

d. A tiny particle with a positive charge that orbits an atom.

**65. What law states that, in a chemical change, energy can be neither created nor destroyed, but only changed from one form to another?**

a. The Law of the Preservation of Matter

b. The Law of the Conservation of Energy

c. The Law of the Conservation of Energy

d. The Law of the Conservation of Energy

**66. What is the simplest unit of any compound?**

a. Atom

b. Proton

c. Molecule

d. Compound

**67. Sex chromosomes are designated as being "X" or "Y" chromosomes. In terms of sex chromosomes, what differences exist between males and females?**

   a. Females have two X chromosomes and males have one X chromosome and one Y chromosome.

   b. Females have one X chromosome, and males have one X chromosome and one Y chromosome.

   c. Females have one Y chromosome, while males have one X chromosome.

   d. Females have one X chromosome and one Y chromosome, and males have two X chromosomes.

**68. A biofilm is**

   a. A dense aggregation of bacteria attached to surfaces.
   b. A type of bacteria which causes disease.
   c. A cluster of bacteria which is healthy to consume.
   d. Bacteria which aids in digestion.

**69. Identify the chemical properties of water.**

   a. Water has two hydrogen atoms covalently bonded to one oxygen atom.
   b. Water has two oxygen atoms covalently bonded to one hydrogen atom.
   c. Water has two hydrogen atoms polar covalently bonded to one oxygen atom.
   d. Water has two oxygen atoms polar covalently bonded to one hydrogen atom.

**70. Which of the following is not true of atomic theory?**

   a. Originated 2500 years ago with Greek philosopher, Leucippus and his pupil Democritus

   b. Is the field of physics that describes the characteristics and properties of atoms that make up matter.

   c. Explains temperature as the momentum of atoms.

   d. Explains macroscopic phenomenon through the behavior of microscopic atoms.

**71. Calculate the molarity of 2.5 liters of a lithium fluoride, LiF solution that contains 52 grams of LiF. (Gram-formula - atomic mass =26 grams/mole)**

   a. 0.8 M
   b. 1.5 M
   c. 0.5 mol
   d. 2 mol

72. In physics, _____ is the force that opposes the relative motion of two bodies in contact.

   a. Resistance
   b. Abrasiveness
   c. Friction
   d. Antagonism

73. What is the difference between anabolism and catabolism?

   a. Anabolism is the series of chemical reactions resulting in the synthesis of inorganic compounds, and catabolism is a series of chemical reactions that break down larger molecules.
   b. Anabolism is the series of chemical reactions resulting in the synthesis of organic compounds, and catabolism is a series of chemical reactions that combine larger molecules.
   c. Catabolism is the series of chemical reactions resulting in the synthesis of organic compounds, and anabolism is a series of chemical reactions that break down larger molecules.
   d. Anabolism is the series of chemical reactions resulting in the synthesis of organic compounds, and catabolism is a series of chemical reactions that break down larger molecules.

74. What results when acid reacts with a base?

   a. A weak acid
   b. A weak base
   c. A salt and water
   d. Hydrogen

75. What is a reaction where an element gains electrons known as?

   a. Reduction
   b. Oxidation
   c. Sublimation
   d. Condensation

# Answer Key

## Section 1 – Verbal Ability

### Part 1 – Reading Comprehension

**1. A**
Helen's parents hired Anne to teach Helen to communicate. Choice B is incorrect because the passage states Anne had trouble finding her way around, which means she could walk. Choice C is incorrect because you don't hire a teacher to teach someone to play. Choice D is incorrect because by age 6, if Helen had never eaten, she would have starved to death.

**2. B**
The correct answer because that fact is stated directly in the passage. The passage explains that Anne taught Helen to hear by allowing her to feel the vibrations in her throat.

**3. A**
We can infer that Anne is a patient teacher because she did not leave or lose her temper when Helen bit or hit her; she just kept trying to teach Helen. Choice B is incorrect because Anne taught Helen to read and talk. Choice C is incorrect because Anne could hear. She was partially blind, not deaf. Choice D is incorrect because it does not have to do with patience.

**4. B**
The passage states that it was hard for anyone but Anne to understand Helen when she spoke. Choice A is incorrect because the passage does not mention Helen spoke a foreign language. Choice C is incorrect because there is no mention of how quiet or loud Helen's voice was. Choice D is incorrect because we know from reading the passage that Helen did learn to speak.

**5. D**
This question tests the reader's summarization skills. The question is asking very generally about the message of the passage, and the title, "Ways Characters Communicate in Theater," is one indication of that. The other choices A, B, and C are all directly from the text, and therefore readers may be inclined to select one of them, but are too specific to encapsulate the entirety of the passage and its message.

**6. B**
The paragraph on soliloquies mentions "To be or not to be," and it is from the context of that paragraph that readers may understand that because "To be or not to be" is a soliloquy, Hamlet will be introspective, or thoughtful, while delivering it. It is true that actors deliver soliloquies alone, and may be "solitary" (choice A), but "thoughtful" (choice B) is more true to the overall idea of the paragraph. Readers may choose C because drama and theater can be used interchangeably and the passage mentions that soliloquies are unique to theater (and therefore drama), but this answer is not specific enough to the paragraph in question. Readers may pick up on the theme of life and death and Hamlet's true intentions and select that he is "hopeless" (choice D), but those themes are not discussed either by this paragraph or passage, as a close textual reading and analysis confirms.

**7. C**
This question tests the reader's grammatical skills. Choice B seems logical, but parenthesis are actually considered to be a stronger break in a sentence than commas are, and along this line of thinking, actually disrupt the sentence more.

Choices A and D make comparisons between theater and film that are not made in the passage, and may or may not be true. This detail does clarify the statement that asides are most unique to theater by adding that it is not completely unique to theater, which may have been why the author didn't chose not to delete it and instead used parentheses to designate the detail's importance (choice C).

**8. A**
Low blood sugar occurs both in diabetics and healthy adults.

**9. B**
None of the statements are the author's opinion.

**10. A**
The author's purpose is the inform.

**11. A**
The only statement that is not a detail is, "A doctor can diagnosis this medical condition by asking the patient questions and testing."

**12. A**
This sentence is a recommendation.

**13. C**
Tips for a good night's sleep is the best alternative title for this article.

**14. B**
Mental activity is helpful for a good night's sleep is cannot be inferred from this article.

**15. A**
From the passage, one disadvantage of taking naps is they may keep you awake at night.

**16. C**
Based on the partial table of contents, you would find information about natural selection in the ecology section on page 110.

**17. C**
To be infamous means to be remembered for an evil or terrible action. Therefore, the word infamy means to remember a bad or terrible thing. Choice A is incorrect because being famous is not the same as being infamous. Choice B is incorrect because the attack on Pearl Harbor was not good. Choice D is incorrect because Pearl Harbor was not forgotten.

**18. C**
Each answer choice except choice C contains the name of at least one country that was not part of the AXIS powers.

**19. D**
It is stated in the passage. Choice A is not correct because there was no indication that Japan would attack San Diego. Choice B is incorrect because the attack on Pearl Harbor was a surprise. Choice C is incorrect because Roosevelt was not planning to attack Japan.

**20. C**
The passage clearly states that Japan planned a surprise attack. They chose that early time to catch the U.S. military off guard. Choice A is incorrect because the military does not sleep late. Choice B is incorrect because there is no law against bombing countries. Choice D is incorrect because it makes no sense.

**21. C**
This question tests the reader's vocabulary skills. The uses of the negatives "but" and "less," especially right next to each other, may confuse readers into answering with choices A or D, which list words that are antonyms to "militant." Readers may also be confused by the comparison of healthy people with what is being described as an overly healthy person--both people are good, but the reader may look for which one is "worse" in the comparison, and therefore stray toward the antonym words. One key to understanding the meaning of "militant" if the reader is unfamiliar with it is to look at the root of the word; readers can then easily associate it with "military" and gain a sense of what the word signifies: defence (especially considered that the immune system defends the body).

Choice C is correct over choice B because "militant" is an adjective, just as the words in choice C are, whereas the words in choice B are nouns.

**22. C**
This question tests the reader's understanding of function within writing. The other choices are details included surrounding the quoted text, and may therefore confuse the reader. A somewhat contradicts what is said earlier in the paragraph, which is that tests and treatments are improving, and probably doctors are along with them, but the paragraph doesn't actually mention doctors, and the subject of the question is the medicine. Choice B may seem correct to readers who aren't careful to understand that, while the author does mention the large number of people effected, the author is touching on the realities of living with allergies, rather than the likelihood of curing all allergies. Similarly, while the author does mention the "balance" of the body, which is easily associated with "wholesome," the author is not really making an argument and especially is not making an extreme statement that allergy medicines should be outlawed. Again, because the article's tone is on living with allergies, choice C is an appropriate choice that fits with the title and content of the text.

**23. B**
This question tests the reader's inference skills. The text does not state who is doing the recommending, but the use of the "patients," as well as the general context of the passage, lends itself to the logical partner, "doctors," choice B. The author does mention the recommendation but doesn't present it as her own (i.e. "I recommend that"), so choice A may be eliminated. It may seem plausible that people with allergies (choice D) may recommend medicines or products to other people with allergies, but the text does not necessarily support this interaction taking place. Choice C may be selected because the EpiPen is specifically mentioned, but the use of the phrase "such as" when it is introduced is not limiting enough to assume the recommendation is coming from its creators.

**24. D**
This question tests the reader's global understanding of the text. Choice D includes the main topics of the three body paragraphs, and isn't too focused on a specific aspect or quote from the text, as the other questions are, giving a skewed summary of what the author intended. The reader may be drawn to choice B because of the title of the passage and the use of words like "better," but the message of the passage is larger and more general than this.

**25. B**
Reading the document posted to the Human Resources website is optional.

**26. B**
The document is recommended changes and have not be implemented yet.

**27. C**
This question tests the reader's summarization skills. The use of the word "actually" in describing what kind of people poets are, as well as other moments like this, may lead readers to selecting choices B or D, but the author is more information than trying to persuade readers. The author gives no indication that she loves poetry (choice B) or that people, students specifically (D), should write poems. Choice A is incorrect because the style and content of this paragraph do not match those of a foreword; forewords usually focus on the history or ideas of a specific poem to introduce it more fully and help it stand out against other poems. The author here focuses on several poems and gives broad statements. Instead, she tells a kind of story about poems, giving three very broad time periods in which to discuss them, thereby giving a brief history of poetry, as choice C states.

**28. A**
This question tests the reader's summarization skills. Key words in the topic sentences of each of the paragraphs ("oldest," "Renaissance," "modern") should give the reader an idea that the author is moving chronologically. The opening and closing sentence-paragraphs are broad and talk generally. B seems reasonable, but epic poems are mentioned in two paragraphs, eliminating the idea that only new types of poems are used in each paragraph. Choice C is also easily eliminated because the author clearly mentions several different poets, groups of people, and poems. Choice D also seems reasonable, considering that the author does move from older forms of poetry to newer forms, but use of "so (that)" makes this statement false, for the author gives no indication that she is rushing (the paragraphs are about the same size) or that she prefers modern poetry.

**29. D**
This question tests the reader's attention to detail. The key word is "invented"--it ties together the Mesopotamians, who invented the written word, and the fact that they, as the inventors, also invented and used poetry. The other selections focus on other details mentioned in the passage, such as that the Renaissance's admiration of the Greeks (choice C) and that Beowulf is in Old English (choice A). Choice B may seem like an attractive answer because it is unlike the others and because the idea of heroes seems rooted in ancient and early civilizations.

**30. B**
This question tests the reader's vocabulary and contextualization skills. "Telling" is not an unusual word, but it may be used here in a way that is not familiar to readers, as an adjective rather than a verb in gerund form. Choice A may seem like the obvious answer to a reader looking for a verb to match the use they are familiar with. If the reader understands that the word is being used as an adjective and that choice A is a ploy, they may opt to select choice D, "wordy," but it does not make sense in context. Choice C can be easily eliminated, and doesn't have any connection to the paragraph or passage. "Significant" (choice B) makes sense contextually, especially relative to the phrase "give insight" used later in the sentence.

## Verbal Ability Part II - Vocabulary

**31. C**
**Dauntless:** adj. Invulnerable to fear or intimidation.

**32. A**
**Juxtaposed:** adj. Placed side-by-side, often for comparison or contrast.

**33. B**
**Regicide:** v. killing of a king.

**34. A**
**Pernicious:** adj. Causing much harm in a subtle way.

**35. A**
**Immune:** adj. Resistant to a particular infection or toxin owing to the presence of specific antibodies.

**36. B**
**Nimble:** adj. Quick and light in movement or action.

**37. A**
**Queries:** n. Questions or inquiries.

**38. C**
**Depose:** To remove (a leader) from (high) office, without killing the incumbent.

**39. D**
**Pedestrian:** Ordinary, dull; everyday; unexceptional.

**40. B**
**Petulant:** adj. Childishly irritable.

**41. D**
**Pesticide:** n. A substance used for destroying insects or other organisms harmful to cultivated plants or to animals.

**42. D**
**Salient:** adj. worthy or note or relevant.

**43. B**
**Sedentary:** adj. not moving or sitting in one place.

**44. A**
**Famine:** n. extreme scarcity of food.

**45. A**
**Stint:** n. To be sparing.

**46. A**
**Precipitate:** v. to rain.

**47. C**
**Edify:** v. To instruct or improve morally or intellectually.

**48. B**
**Egress:** n. An exit or way out.

**49. A**
**Recede:** v. To move back, to move away.

**50. A**
**Confidential:** adj. kept secret within a certain circle of persons; not intended to be known publicly.

**51. A**
**Aggravate:** v. to make worse, or more severe; to render less tolerable or less excusable; to make more offensive; to enhance; to intensify.

**52. B**
**Debut:** n. a performer's first-time performance to the public.

**53. B**
**Hormones:** n. A regulatory substance produced in an organism and transported in tissue fluids such as blood or sap to stimulate specific cells.

**54. B**
**Importune:** v. To harass with persistent requests.

**55. B**
**Sedulous:** adj. Showing dedication and diligence.

**56. A**
**Tincture:** n. alcoholic drink with plant extracts used for medicine.

**57. C**
**Felony:** n. Serious criminal offence that is punishable by death or imprisonment above a year.

**58. A**
**Bibliophile**: n. One who loves books.

**59. A**
**Monsoons:** n. The rainy season accompanying the wet monsoon.

**60. D**
**Volatile:** adj. Explosive.

## Section II – Mathematics

**1. A**
1/3 X 3/4 = 3/12 = 1/4

**2. D**
75/1500 = 15/300 = 3/60 = 1/20

**3. B**

We remove the brackets and we group the variables by degrees.

$-4x^2 + x + 5$

$(-3x^2 + 2x + 6) + (-x^2 - x - 1) =$

$-3x^2 + 2x + 6 - x^2 - x - 1 =$

$-4x^2 + x + 5$

**4. D**
3.14 + 2.73 = 5.87 and 5.87 + 23.7 = 29.57

**5. D**
First add all the numbers 200,000 + 10,020 + 30,000 + 15,000 + 1080 = 256,100. Then divide by 5 (the number of data provided) = 256,100/5 = 51,220

**6. C**
0.27 + 0.33 = 0.6 = 60/100 = 3/5.

**7. D**
3.13 + 7.87 = 11 and 11 X 5 = 55

**8. A**
3 x 3 x 3 x 3 = 81

**9. B**
2/4 X 3/4 = 6/16, in lowest terms = 3/8

**10. D**
$2(5)^3 - (2)^3 = 2(125) - 8 = 250 - 8 = 242$

**11. C**
3/10 * 90 = 3 * 90/10 = 270/10 = 27

**12. C**
First add all the numbers 1 + 2 + 3 + 4 + 5 +6 + 7 +8 + 9 + 10 = 55. Then divide by 10 (the number of data provided) = 55/5 = 11

**13. B**
.4/100 * 36 = .4 * 36/100 = 14.4/100 = 0.144

**14. D**
To solve for x,
5x – 7x + 3 = -1
5x – 7x = -1 -3
-2x = -4
x = -4/ -2
x = 2

**15. B**
There are two statements made. This means that we can write two equations according to these statements:
The sum of two numbers are 21: x + y = 21

The sum of the squares is 261: $x^2 + y^2 = 261$

We are asked to find x and y.

Since we have the sums of the numbers and the sums of their squares; we can use the square formula of x + y, that is:

$(x + y)^2 = x^2 + 2xy + y^2$ ... Here, we can insert the known values x + y and $x^2 + y^2$:

$(21)^2 = 261 + 2xy$ ... Arranging to find xy:

441 = 261 + 2xy

441 - 261 = 2xy

180 = 2xy

xy = 180/2

xy = 90

We need to find two number which multiply to 90. Checking the answer choices, we see that in (b), 15 and 6 are given. 15•6 = 90. Also their squares sum up to 261 ($15^2 + 6^2$ = 225 + 36 = 261). So these two numbers satisfy the equation.

**16. C**
To solve for x, first simplify the equation
$5x + 2x + 14 = 14x - 7$
$7x + 14 = 14x - 7$
$7x - 14x + 14 = -7$
$7x - 14x = -7 - 14$
$-7x = -21$
$x = -21/-7$
$x = 3$

**17. C**
$5z + 5 = 3z + 6 + 11$
$5z - 3z + 5 = 6 + 11$
$5z - 3z = 6 + 11 - 5$
$2z = 17 - 5$
$2z = 12$
$z = 12/2$
$z = 6$

**18. C**
To make this easier break 81 to 9 x 9 and then find the prime factors of each of these prime numbers. The prime factors of 9 = 3 x 3 and the prime factors of 9 = 3 x 3
Prime factors of 81 = 3 x 3 x 3 x 3

**19. D**
Price increased by $5 ($25-$20). The percent increase is 5/20 x 100 = 5 x 5 = 25%

**20. D**
30/100 x 150 = 3 x 15 = 45 (increase in number of correct answers). So the number of correct answers in second test will be the number of correct answers in the first test plus the increase, which is, 150 + 45 = 195

**21. C**
(4 x 4 x 4) + (2 x 2 x 2 x 2) = 64 + 16 = 80

**22. D**
As the lawn is square, the length of one side will be the square root of the area. √62,500 = 250 meters. So, the perimeter is found by 4 times the length of the side of the square:

250 * 4 = 1000 meters.

Since each meter costs $5.5, the total cost of the fence will be 1000•5.5 = $5,500.

**23. C**
p = 1.5 x 18 = 27 kg x m/s into the field.

**24. D**
The decimal point moves 2 spaces right to be placed after 2, which is the first non-zero number. Thus it is $2.04 \times 10^2$

**25. B**
There are 50 balls in the basket now. Let x be the number of yellow balls that are to be added to make 65%. So the equation becomes
X + 15 /X + 50 = 65/100
X = 50

**26. C**
There are 144 students and each bus holds 36, so 144/36 = 4 buses.

**27. D**
$x^2 + 4x + 4 = 0$ ... We try to separate the middle term 4x to find common factors with $x^2$ and 4 separately:

$x^2 + 2x + 2x + 4 = 0$ ... Here, we see that x is a common factor for $x^2$ and 2x, and 2 is a common factor for 2x and 4:

$x(x + 2) + 2(x + 2) = 0$ ... Here, we have x times x + 2 and 2 times x + 2 summed up. This means that we have x + 2 times x + 2:

$(x + 2)(x + 2) = 0$

$(x + 2)^2 = 0$ ... This is true if only if x + 2 is equal to zero.

$x + 2 = 0$

$x = -2$

**28. C**
The sum of angles around a point is 360°
d + 300 = 360°
d = 60°

**29. A**
The wheel travels 2πr distance when it makes one revolution. Here, r stands for the radius. The radius is given as 25 cm in the figure. So,

2πr = 2π * 25 = 50π cm is the distance traveled in one revolution.

In 175 revolutions: 175 * 50π = 8750π cm is traveled.

We are asked to find the distance in meter.

1 m = 100 cm So;

8750π cm = 8750π / 100 = 87.5π m

**30. C**
Pythagorean Theorem:
$(Hypotenuse)^2 = (Perpendicular)^2 + (Base)^2$
$h^2 = a^2 + b^2$

Given: $3^2 + 4^2 = h^2$
$h^2 = 9 + 16$
$h = \sqrt{25}$
$h = 5$

**31. D**
Shaded area= Outer area – Inner area(square + rectangle)
Shaded area= (8 x 8) –{(2 x 2) + [(3 + 2) x 4]}, = 64 – (4 + 20), =
64- 24
Shaded area= 40 cm²

**32. A**
Black stone for 200 tiles = 200 x [Total tile area – Inner white area(4 triangles)]
= 200 x [(162)-(4x1/2 x 8 x 8)] = 200 x (256-128) = 200 x 128 = 25600 cm²
Converting to meters – 1 cm. = 0.01 meters
= 25600/100 m²
= 256 m²

**33. B**
If we know the coordinates of two points on a line, we can find the slope (m) with the below formula:

$m = (y_2 - y_1)/(x_2 - x_1)$ where $(x_1, y_1)$ represent the coordinates of one point and $(x_2, y_2)$ the other.

In this question:

$(-4, -4) : x_1 = -4, y_1 = -4$

$(-1, 2) : x_2 = -1, y_2 = 2$

Inserting these values into the formula:

m = (2 - (-4))/(-1 - (-4)) = (2 + 4)/(-1 + 4) = 6/3 ... Simplifying by 3:

m = 2

**34. A**
The equation for the total liters of wine will be y = 0.20x + 2

**35. C**
If it takes 12 men to operate four machines, then, 12 is to 4, as X is to 20. So X must be 3 X 20 = 60.

**36. C**
If there are 5 friends and each drink costs $1.89, we can round up to $2 per drink and estimate the total cost at, 5 X $2 = $10.

The actual cost is 5 X $1.89 = $9.45.

**37. D**
First convert 500g to kg = 500/1000 = 0.5kg, momentum = 0.5 x 3.5 = 1.75 kg x m/s along the road

**38. A**
$\sqrt{121}$

**39. D**
The smallest prime number that can divide 25 is 5. 25/5 = 5. Prime factors of 25 = 5 x 5

**40. D**
The decimal point moves 5 places left to be placed after 2, which is the first non-zero number. Thus its 2.011 x $10^{-5}$ The answer is in the negative because the decimal moved left

**41. D**
7: 25 =X:100
25/7 = 3.5
100/3.5 = 28.5

**42. B**
The relation is two upright figures in the first set, and 2 horizontal figures in the second set.

**43. C**
The first pair contains a box with a circle inside, and the same figure on its side.

**44. C**
The inside and larger shapes are reversed.

**45. B**
$6x^2 - 5$
$3x^3 + 2x^2 + 5x - 7 + 4x^2 - 5x + 2 - 3x^3 = 6x^2 - 5$

**46. B**
Formula for volume of a shape is L x W x H = 15 x 20 x 10 = 3,000m³

**47. A**
465,890 - 456,890 = 9,000

**48. C**
3/4 + 2/4 + 1.2, first convert the decimal to fraction, = 3/4 + 2/4 + 1 1/5 = ¾ + 2/4 + 6/5 = (find common denominator) (15 + 10 + 24)/20 = 49/20 = 2 9/20

**49. D**
1 inch on map = 2,000 inches on ground. So, 5.2 inches on map = 5.2 * 2,000 = 10,400 inches on ground.

**50. C**
The ratio of black balls to white is 38:42. Reduce to lowest terms = 19:21

## Section III – Science

**1. A**
The formula for acceleration = A = $(V_f - V_0)/t$
So A = (120 -90)/5 sec = 6 mph/second²

**2. A**
Only genetics pertains directly to the cell's function. For genetics, the cell of a new organism acquires traits of ancestral organisms.

**3. A**
A solution with a pH value of greater than 7 is base.

**4. B**
The voltage across a resistor is equal to the product of the resistance and the current flowing through it.

**5. D**
Both have single membrane compartments.

**6. C**
Electric potential is a fundamental interaction between the magnetic field and the presence and motion of an electric charge.

Electric potential is the capacity of an electric field to do work on an electric charge, typically measured in volts, while electromagnetism is a fundamental interaction between the magnetic field and the presence and motion of an electric charge.

**7. C**
Subversion. Active transport, adhesion and cell signaling are all involved in cellular biology.

**8. C**
Homologous is being inherited by the organisms' common ancestors. An example would be feathers and hair—both share a common ancestral trait.

**9. C**
The manner in which instructions for building proteins, the basic structural molecules of living material are written in the DNA is a **genetic code**.

**10. C**
A gene is a unit of inherited material, encoded by a strand of DNA and transcribed by RNA.

**11. B**
Speed = (total distance traveled)/(total time taken)
6 = x/120   (convert minutes to seconds)
6 * 120 = x
X = 720 meters

**12. D**
Cellular scientists' biographies are not studied in cell biology. The physiological properties of cells, cell structure and the life cycle of a cell are all valid topics of study within cell biology.

**13. A**
Detection of pathogens can be complicated because they evolve so quickly.

**14. C**
Molarity = moles of solute/liters of solution = 8/4 = 2

**15. D**
An ohm ($\Omega$) is a unit of electrical voltage is not true.

**Note:** An ohm is a unit of electrical resistance.

**16. D**
The periodic table contains 118 elements.

**17. C**
Mutations in DNA sequences usually occur spontaneously is false.

**18. C**
Momentum is a product of velocity and mass. If they are all traveling at the same speed, the car that weighs the most would have the highest momentum.

**19. A**
Starting with the weakest, the fundamental forces of nature in order of strength are, Gravity, Weak nuclear force, Electromagnetic force, Strong nuclear force.

**20. A**
Electrons are subatomic particles that carry a negative charge.

**21. A**
Cell culture is the technique for growing cells independent of a living organism within the confines of a laboratory. The cell culture is generally grown in a test-tube environment or on a petri dish.

**22. A**
Precision, which refers to the repeatability of measurement, does not require knowledge of the correct or true value.

**23. A**
Force = Mass times Acceleration Measured in Newtons.
F = 2000 kg X 3 m/sec$^2$ = 6000 N

**24. B**
The periodic table is a tabular display of the chemical elements, organized on the basis of their atomic numbers, electron configurations, and recurring chemical properties.

**25. D**
The scientific discipline that studies the physiological aspects, structures, life cycles and division of cells is called cell biology.

**26. A**
Ionization energy is the minimum amount of energy required to remove an electron from an atom or ion in the gas phase.

**27. C**
Redox is a complete reaction comprising oxidation and reduction reactions that are each only half of the complete reaction. The same exact electrons lost in oxidation are what are gained in reduction.

**28. A**
In terms of the scientific method, the term **observation** refers to the act of noticing or perceiving something and/or recording a fact or occurrence.

**29. B**
The Lewis Theory defines acids and bases in terms of the electron-pair concept; according to its definition, an acid is an electron-pair acceptor, and a base is an electron-pair donor.

**30. A**
First convert 250 ml to liters, 250/1000 = 0.25 then calculate molarity = 5 moles/ 0.25 liters = 20 M.

**31. D**
The property of a conductor that restricts its internal flow of electrons is resistance.

**32. A**
Prokaryotic microorganisms that are usually just a few micrometers long.

**33. B**
Kinetic energy is the energy of a body that results from motion while potential energy is the energy possessed by an object by virtue of its position or state, e.g., as in a compressed spring.

**34. B**
The formula for acceleration = A = $(V_f - V_0)/t$
So A = (2000 - 0)/25 sec = 80 m/sec$^2$

**35. A**
The four states in which matter exists are solid, fluid, gas, and plasma.
The state of matter is determined by the strength of the bonds between the atoms that make up matter.

**36. A**
The cell membrane is a biological membrane that separates the interior of all cells from the outside environment. The cell membrane is selectively permeable to ions and organic molecules and controls the movement of substances in and out of cells.

**37. C**
Electric current is the flow of electric charge through a medium.

**38. D**
Cubes rarely occur naturally, especially in the micro world outside the human eye. True cubes are usually deliberately created.

**39. D**
All acids contain hydrogen. When acids react with most metals, the metals displace the hydrogen and hydrogen gas is produced.

**40. D**
Relative position. Ranks include Domain, Kingdom, Phylum, Class, Order, Family, Genus, and Species.

**41. B**
The following statements about the periodic table of the elements is true,
The way in which the elements are arranged allows for predictions to made about their behavior.

**42. D**
The scientific term **experiment** refers to a practical test designed with the intention that its results be relevant to a particular theory or set of theories.

**43. B**
Substances that deactivate catalysts are called catalytic poisons.

**44. B**
Atmospheric pressure is the force per unit area exerted against a surface by the weight of air above that surface in the Earth's atmosphere.

**45. B**
Kinetic energy is the energy an object possesses due to its motion.

**46. D**
Scientific classification. The two phrases are interchangeable, although the former seems to more accurately reflect the purpose of classification: to categorize biological units.

**47. D**
Oxidation and reduction reactions are each just half of a redox reaction and both occur simultaneously, because the exact electrons lost in oxidation is what is gained in reduction.

**48. C**
A recessive gene is not expressed as a trait unless inherited by both parents.

**49. D**
A **scientific model** is an approximation or simulation of a real system that omits all but the most essential variables of the system.

**50. A**
$X/4.5 = 1.5$, $X = 4.5/1.5 = 3$ mol.

**51. A**
Neutrons are necessary within an atomic nucleus as they bind with protons via the nuclear force.

**52. A**
Atoms of different elements combine in simple whole-number ratios to form chemical compounds.

**53. C**
The following statement is false - Most enzymes are inorganic.

**54. C**
**Acids** are compounds that contain hydrogen and can dissolve in water to release hydrogen ions into solution.

**55. B**
Formula - $P = kg \times m/s$
$= 12.05 kg \times 8 m/s$
$= 96.4 \ kg \times m/s$ down the hill.

Note that the final answer has the proper SI unit of momentum (kg x m/s) after it and it also mentions the direction of the movement.

**56. D**
All of the statements are true.

    a. A non-metal is a substance that conducts heat and electricity poorly.

    b. Most of the known chemical elements are non-metals.

    c. A non-metal is brittle or waxy or gaseous.

**57. B**
The discipline that studies bacteria is Bacteriology.

**58. A**
Genes determine individual hereditary characteristics.

**59. C**
A and B are true.

    a. Light consists of electromagnetic waves in the visible range.

    b. The fundamental particle or quantum of light is a photon.

**Note:** Light energy is the only visible form of energy. A light bulb is a device that uses electrical energy to create electromagnetic energy in the form (in part) of visible light and heat.

**60. A**
The groups into which organisms are classified are called taxa and include, in order of size, Genus, Kingdom, Phylum/division, Class, Order, and Family Species.

**61. A**
Chemical bonds are attractions between atoms that form chemical substances containing two or more atoms.

**62. C**
In chemistry, the number of protons in the nucleus of an atom is known as the atomic number, which determines the chemical element to which the atom belongs.

**63. D**
The molarity of an aqueous solution of CaCl is defined as the moles of CaCl per liter of solution.

**64. C**
An electron is a tiny particle with a negative charge that orbits a nucleus.

**65. C**
The Law of the Conservation of Energy states that, in a chemical change, energy can be neither created nor destroyed, but only changed from one form to another.

**66. A**
An atom is the basic or fundamental unit of any matter or element.

**67. A**
Females have two X chromosomes and males have one X chromosome and one Y chromosome.

**68. A**
A biofilm is a dense aggregation of bacteria attached to surfaces. The density of these bacteria is based on many factors, such as environment, temperature, and how long they are left undisturbed.

**69. A**
Water has two hydrogen atoms covalently bonded to one oxygen atom.

**70. C**
Choice C (Atomic theory explains temperature as the momentum of atoms) is incorrect because atomic theory explains temperature as the motion of atoms (faster = hotter), not the momentum. The momentum of atoms explains the outward pressure that they exert.

**71. A**
First convert LiF grams to moles = 52 x 1/26 = 2. Now Molarity = 2 moles/2.5 liters = 0.8 M

**72. C**
In physics, friction is the force that opposes the relative motion of two bodies in contact.

**73. D**
Anabolism is the series of chemical reactions resulting in the synthesis of organic compounds, and catabolism is a series of chemical reactions that break down larger molecules.

**74. C**
When an acid and a base react, they neutralize each other's properties to form salt and water.

**75. A**
Reduction is a reaction that usually involves the gain of electrons that were lost in an oxidation reaction.

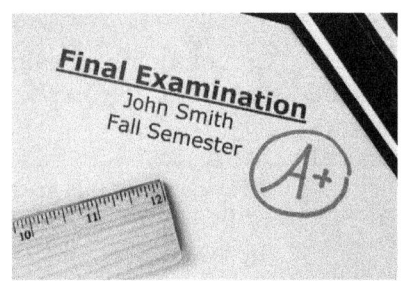

# Practice Test Questions Set 2

The questions below are not the same as you will find on the PAX RN - that would be too easy! And nobody knows what the questions will be and they change all the time. Below are general questions that cover the same subject areas as the PAX RN. So while the format and exact wording of the questions may differ slightly, and change from year to year, if you can answer the questions below, you will have no problem with the PAX RN.

For the best results, take this Practice Test as if it were the real exam. Set aside time when you will not be disturbed, and a location that is quiet and free of distractions. Read the instructions carefully, read each question carefully, and answer to the best of your ability.

Use the bubble answer sheets provided. When you have completed the Practice Test, check your answer against the Answer Key and read the explanation provided.

Do not attempt more than one set of practice test questions in one day. After completing the first practice test, wait two or three days before attempting the second set of questions.

### Section I – Verbal Ability
**Questions:** 80 **Time:** 60 Minutes

### Section II – Mathematics
**Questions:** 50 **Time:** 60 Minutes

### Section III – Science
**Questions:** 75 **Time:** 60 minutes

# Verbal Ability

1. Ⓐ Ⓑ Ⓒ Ⓓ
2. Ⓐ Ⓑ Ⓒ Ⓓ
3. Ⓐ Ⓑ Ⓒ Ⓓ
4. Ⓐ Ⓑ Ⓒ Ⓓ
5. Ⓐ Ⓑ Ⓒ Ⓓ
6. Ⓐ Ⓑ Ⓒ Ⓓ
7. Ⓐ Ⓑ Ⓒ Ⓓ
8. Ⓐ Ⓑ Ⓒ Ⓓ
9. Ⓐ Ⓑ Ⓒ Ⓓ
10. Ⓐ Ⓑ Ⓒ Ⓓ
11. Ⓐ Ⓑ Ⓒ Ⓓ
12. Ⓐ Ⓑ Ⓒ Ⓓ
13. Ⓐ Ⓑ Ⓒ Ⓓ
14. Ⓐ Ⓑ Ⓒ Ⓓ
15. Ⓐ Ⓑ Ⓒ Ⓓ
16. Ⓐ Ⓑ Ⓒ Ⓓ
17. Ⓐ Ⓑ Ⓒ Ⓓ
18. Ⓐ Ⓑ Ⓒ Ⓓ
19. Ⓐ Ⓑ Ⓒ Ⓓ
20. Ⓐ Ⓑ Ⓒ Ⓓ
21. Ⓐ Ⓑ Ⓒ Ⓓ
22. Ⓐ Ⓑ Ⓒ Ⓓ
23. Ⓐ Ⓑ Ⓒ Ⓓ
24. Ⓐ Ⓑ Ⓒ Ⓓ
25. Ⓐ Ⓑ Ⓒ Ⓓ
26. Ⓐ Ⓑ Ⓒ Ⓓ
27. Ⓐ Ⓑ Ⓒ Ⓓ
28. Ⓐ Ⓑ Ⓒ Ⓓ
29. Ⓐ Ⓑ Ⓒ Ⓓ
30. Ⓐ Ⓑ Ⓒ Ⓓ
31. Ⓐ Ⓑ Ⓒ Ⓓ
32. Ⓐ Ⓑ Ⓒ Ⓓ
33. Ⓐ Ⓑ Ⓒ Ⓓ
34. Ⓐ Ⓑ Ⓒ Ⓓ
35. Ⓐ Ⓑ Ⓒ Ⓓ
36. Ⓐ Ⓑ Ⓒ Ⓓ
37. Ⓐ Ⓑ Ⓒ Ⓓ
38. Ⓐ Ⓑ Ⓒ Ⓓ
39. Ⓐ Ⓑ Ⓒ Ⓓ
40. Ⓐ Ⓑ Ⓒ Ⓓ
41. Ⓐ Ⓑ Ⓒ Ⓓ
42. Ⓐ Ⓑ Ⓒ Ⓓ
43. Ⓐ Ⓑ Ⓒ Ⓓ
44. Ⓐ Ⓑ Ⓒ Ⓓ
45. Ⓐ Ⓑ Ⓒ Ⓓ
46. Ⓐ Ⓑ Ⓒ Ⓓ
47. Ⓐ Ⓑ Ⓒ Ⓓ
48. Ⓐ Ⓑ Ⓒ Ⓓ
49. Ⓐ Ⓑ Ⓒ Ⓓ
50. Ⓐ Ⓑ Ⓒ Ⓓ
51. Ⓐ Ⓑ Ⓒ Ⓓ
52. Ⓐ Ⓑ Ⓒ Ⓓ
53. Ⓐ Ⓑ Ⓒ Ⓓ
54. Ⓐ Ⓑ Ⓒ Ⓓ
55. Ⓐ Ⓑ Ⓒ Ⓓ
56. Ⓐ Ⓑ Ⓒ Ⓓ
57. Ⓐ Ⓑ Ⓒ Ⓓ
58. Ⓐ Ⓑ Ⓒ Ⓓ
59. Ⓐ Ⓑ Ⓒ Ⓓ
60. Ⓐ Ⓑ Ⓒ Ⓓ
61. Ⓐ Ⓑ Ⓒ Ⓓ
62. Ⓐ Ⓑ Ⓒ Ⓓ
63. Ⓐ Ⓑ Ⓒ Ⓓ
64. Ⓐ Ⓑ Ⓒ Ⓓ
65. Ⓐ Ⓑ Ⓒ Ⓓ
66. Ⓐ Ⓑ Ⓒ Ⓓ
67. Ⓐ Ⓑ Ⓒ Ⓓ
68. Ⓐ Ⓑ Ⓒ Ⓓ
69. Ⓐ Ⓑ Ⓒ Ⓓ
70. Ⓐ Ⓑ Ⓒ Ⓓ
71. Ⓐ Ⓑ Ⓒ Ⓓ
72. Ⓐ Ⓑ Ⓒ Ⓓ
73. Ⓐ Ⓑ Ⓒ Ⓓ
74. Ⓐ Ⓑ Ⓒ Ⓓ
75. Ⓐ Ⓑ Ⓒ Ⓓ
76. Ⓐ Ⓑ Ⓒ Ⓓ
77. Ⓐ Ⓑ Ⓒ Ⓓ
78. Ⓐ Ⓑ Ⓒ Ⓓ
79. Ⓐ Ⓑ Ⓒ Ⓓ
80. Ⓐ Ⓑ Ⓒ Ⓓ

## Mathematics

| | | |
|---|---|---|
| 1. A B C D | 18. A B C D | 35. A B C D |
| 2. A B C D | 19. A B C D | 36. A B C D |
| 3. A B C D | 20. A B C D | 37. A B C D |
| 4. A B C D | 21. A B C D | 38. A B C D |
| 5. A B C D | 22. A B C D | 39. A B C D |
| 6. A B C D | 23. A B C D | 40. A B C D |
| 7. A B C D | 24. A B C D | 41. A B C D |
| 8. A B C D | 25. A B C D | 42. A B C D |
| 9. A B C D | 26. A B C D | 43. A B C D |
| 10. A B C D | 27. A B C D | 44. A B C D |
| 11. A B C D | 28. A B C D | 45. A B C D |
| 12. A B C D | 29. A B C D | 46. A B C D |
| 13. A B C D | 30. A B C D | 47. A B C D |
| 14. A B C D | 31. A B C D | 48. A B C D |
| 15. A B C D | 32. A B C D | 49. A B C D |
| 16. A B C D | 33. A B C D | 50. A B C D |
| 17. A B C D | 34. A B C D | |

## Science

1. A B C D
2. A B C D
3. A B C D
4. A B C D
5. A B C D
6. A B C D
7. A B C D
8. A B C D
9. A B C D
10. A B C D
11. A B C D
12. A B C D
13. A B C D
14. A B C D
15. A B C D
16. A B C D
17. A B C D
18. A B C D
19. A B C D
20. A B C D
21. A B C D
22. A B C D
23. A B C D
24. A B C D
25. A B C D
26. A B C D
27. A B C D
28. A B C D
29. A B C D
30. A B C D
31. A B C D
32. A B C D
33. A B C D
34. A B C D
35. A B C D
36. A B C D
37. A B C D
38. A B C D
39. A B C D
40. A B C D
41. A B C D
42. A B C D
43. A B C D
44. A B C D
45. A B C D
46. A B C D
47. A B C D
48. A B C D
49. A B C D
50. A B C D
51. A B C D
52. A B C D
53. A B C D
54. A B C D
55. A B C D
56. A B C D
57. A B C D
58. A B C D
59. A B C D
60. A B C D
61. A B C D
62. A B C D
63. A B C D
64. A B C D
65. A B C D
66. A B C D
67. A B C D
68. A B C D
69. A B C D
70. A B C D
71. A B C D
72. A B C D
73. A B C D
74. A B C D
75. A B C D
76. A B C D
77. A B C D
78. A B C D
79. A B C D
80. A B C D

# Section I - Verbal Ability

**Directions:** The following questions are based on several reading passages. Each passage is followed by a series of questions. Read each passage carefully, and then answer the questions based on it. You may reread the passage as often as you wish. When you have finished answering the questions based on one passage, go right onto the next passage. Choose the best answer based on the information given and implied.

**Questions 1 - 4 refer to the following passage.**

**Passage 1 - The Crusades**

In 1095 Pope Urban II proclaimed the First Crusade with the intent and stated goal to restore Christian access to holy places in and around Jerusalem. Over the next 200 years there were 6 major crusades and numerous minor crusades in the fight for control of the "Holy Land." Historians are divided on the real purpose of the Crusades, some believing that it was part of a purely defensive war against Islamic conquest; some see them as part of a long-running conflict at the frontiers of Europe; and others see them as confident, aggressive, papal-led expansion attempts by Western Christendom. The impact of the crusades was profound, and judgment of the Crusaders ranges from laudatory to highly critical. However, all agree that the Crusades and wars waged during those crusades were brutal and often bloody. Several hundred thousand Roman Catholic Christians joined the Crusades, they were Christians from all over Europe.

Europe at the time was under the Feudal System, so, while the Crusaders made vows to the Church, they also were beholden to their Feudal Lords. This led to the Crusaders not only fighting the Saracen, the commonly used word for Muslim at the time, but also each other for power and economic gain in the Holy Land. This infighting between the Crusaders is why many historians hold the view that the Crusades were simply a front for Europe to invade the Holy Land for economic gain in the name of the Church. Another factor contributing to this theory is that while the army of crusaders marched towards Jerusalem they pillaged the land as they went. The church and feudal Lords vowing to return the land to its original beauty, and inhabitants, this rarely happened though, as the Lords often kept the land for themselves. A full 800 years after the Crusades, Pope John Paul II expressed his sorrow for the massacre of innocent people and the lasting damage that the Medieval church caused.

**1. What is the tone of this article?**

    a. Subjective

    b. Objective

    c. Persuasive

    d. None of the Above

**2. What can all historians agree on concerning the Crusades?**

    a. It achieved great things

    b. It stabilized the Holy Land

    c. It was bloody and brutal

    d. It helped defend Europe from the Byzantine Empire

**3. What impact did the feudal system have on the Crusades?**

    a. It unified the Crusaders

    b. It helped gather volunteers

    c. It had no effect on the Crusades

    d. It led to infighting, causing more damage than good

**4. What does Saracen mean?**

    a. Muslim

    b. Christian

    c. Knight

    d. Holy Land

**Questions 5 - 8 refer to the following passage.**

**ABC Electric Warranty**

ABC Electric Company warrants that its products are free from defects in material and workmanship. Subject to the conditions and limitations set forth below, ABC Electric will, at its option, either repair or replace any part of its products that prove defective due to improper workmanship or materials.

This limited warranty does not cover any damage to the product from improper installation, accident, abuse, misuse, natural disaster, insufficient or excessive electrical supply, abnormal mechanical or environmental conditions, or any unauthorized disassembly, repair, or modification.

This limited warranty also does not apply to any product on which the original identification information has been altered, or removed, has not been handled or packaged correctly, or has been sold as second-hand.

This limited warranty covers only repair, replacement, refund or credit for defective ABC Electric products, as provided above.

**5. I tried to repair my ABC Electric blender, but could not, so can I get it repaired under this warranty?**

    a. Yes, the warranty still covers the blender

    b. No, the warranty does not cover the blender

    c. Uncertain. ABC Electric may or may not cover repairs under this warranty

**6. My ABC Electric fan is not working. Will ABC Electric provide a new one or repair this one?**

    a. ABC Electric will repair my fan

    b. ABC Electric will replace my fan

    c. ABC Electric could either replace or repair my fan can request either a replacement or a repair.

**7. My stove was damaged in a flood. Does this warranty cover my stove?**

    a. Yes, it is covered.

    b. No, it is not covered.

    c. It may or may not be covered.

    d. ABC Electric will decide if it is covered

**8. Which of the following is an example of improper workmanship?**

    a. Missing parts

    b. Defective parts

    c. Scratches on the front

    d. None of the above

**Questions 9 – 12 refer to the following passage.**

**Passage 2 - Women and Advertising**

Only in the last few generations have media messages been so widespread and so readily seen, heard, and read by so many people. Advertising is an important part of both selling and buying anything from soap to cereal to jeans. For whatever reason, more consumers are women than are men. Media message are subtle but powerful, and more attention has been paid lately to how these message affect women.
Of all the products that women buy, makeup, clothes, and other stylistic or cosmetic products are among the most popular. This means that companies focus their advertising on women, promising them that their product will make her feel, look, or smell better than the next company's product will. This competition has resulted in advertising that is more and more ideal and less and less possible for everyday women. Howev-

er, because women do look to these ideals and the products they represent as how they can potentially become, many women have developed unhealthy attitudes about themselves when they have failed to become those ideals.

In recent years, more companies have tried to change advertisements to be healthier for women. This includes featuring models of more sizes and addressing a huge outcry against unfair tools such as airbrushing and photo editing. There is debate about what the right balance between real and ideal is, because fashion is also considered art and some changes are made to elevate fashionable products purposefully and signify that they are creative, innovative, and the work of individual people. Artists want their freedom protected as much as women do, and advertising agencies are often caught in the middle.

Some claim that the companies who make these changes are not doing enough. Many people worry that there are still not enough models of different sizes and different ethnicities. Some people claim that companies use this healthier type of advertisement not for the good of women, but because they would like to sell products to the women who are looking for these kinds of messages. This is also a hard balance to find: companies need to make money, and women need to feel respected.

While the focus of this change has been on women, advertising can also affect men, and this change will hopefully be a lesson on media for all consumers.

**9. The second paragraph states that advertising focuses on women**

    a. to shape what the ideal should be

    b. because women buy makeup

    c. because women are easily persuaded

    d. because of the types of products that women buy

**10. According to the passage, fashion artists and female consumers are at odds because**

    a. there is a debate going on and disagreement drives people apart

    b. both of them are trying to protect their freedom to do something

    c. artists want to elevate their products above the reach of women

    d. women are creative, innovative, individual people

**11. The author uses the phrase "for whatever reason" in this passage to**

    a. keep the focus of the paragraph on media messages and not on the differences between men and women

    b. show that the reason for this is unimportant

    c. argue that it is stupid that more women are consumers than men

    d. show that he or she is tired of talking about why media messages are important

**12. This passage suggests that**

    a. advertising companies are still working on making their messages better

    b. all advertising companies seek to be more approachable for women

    c. women are only buying from companies that respect them

    d. artists could stop producing fashionable products if they feel bullied

**Questions 13 - 16 refer to the following passage.**

**FDR, the Treaty of Versailles, and the Fourteen Points**

At the conclusion of World War I, those who had won the war and those who were forced to admit defeat welcomed the end of the war and expected that a peace treaty would be signed. The American president, Franklin D. Roosevelt, played an important part in proposing what the agreements should be and did so through his Fourteen Points.
World War I had begun in 1914 when an Austrian archduke was assassinated, leading to a domino effect that pulled the world's most powerful countries into war on a large scale. The war catalysed the creation and use of deadly weapons that had not previously existed, resulting in a great loss of soldiers on both sides of the fighting. More than 9 million soldiers were killed.

The United States agreed to enter the war right before it ended, and many believed that its decision to become finally involved brought on the end of the war. FDR made it very clear that the U.S. was entering the war for moral reasons and had an agenda focused on world peace. The Fourteen Points were individual goals and ideas (focused on peace, free trade, open communication, and self-reliance) that FDR wanted the power nations to strive for now that the war had ended. He was optimistic and had many ideas about what could be accomplished through, and during the post-war peace. However, FDR's fourteen points were poorly received when he presented them to the leaders of other world powers, many of whom wanted only to help their own countries and to punish the Germans for fueling the war, and they fell by the wayside. World War II was imminent, for Germany lost everything.

Some historians believe that the other leaders who participated in the Treaty of Versailles weren't receptive to the Fourteen Points because World War I was fought almost entirely on European soil, and the United States lost much less than did the other powers. FDR was in a unique position to determine the fate of the war, but doing it on his own terms did not help accomplish his goals. This is only one historical example of how the United State has tried to use its power as an important country, but found itself limited because of geological or ideological factors.

**13. The main idea of this passage is that**

a. World War I was unfair because no fighting took place in America

b. World War II happened because of the Treaty of Versailles

c. the power the United States has to help other countries also prevents it from helping other countries

d. Franklin D. Roosevelt was one of the United States' smartest presidents

**14. According to the second paragraph, World War I started because**

a. an archduke was assassinated

b. weapons that were more deadly had been developed

c. a domino effect of allies agreeing to help one another

d. the world's most powerful countries were large

**15. The author includes the detail that 9 million soldiers were killed**

a. to demonstrate why European leaders were hesitant to accept peace

b. to show the reader the dangers of deadly weapons

c. to make the reader think about which countries lost the most soldiers

d. to demonstrate why World War II was imminent

**16. According to this passage, catalysed means**

a. Analyzed

b. Sped up

c. Invented

d. Funded

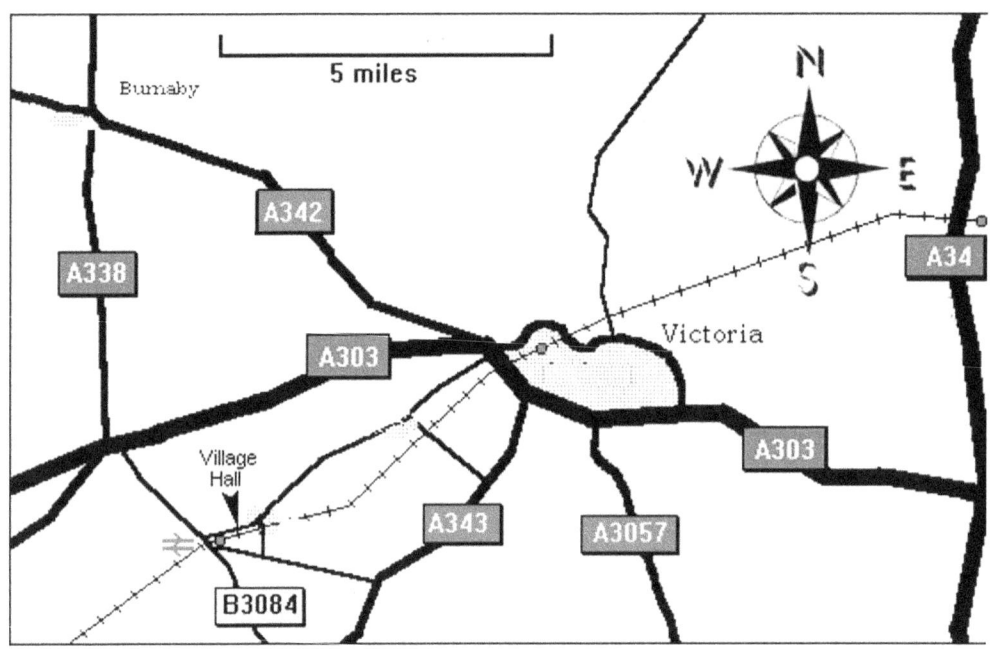

**17. Approximately how far is Victoria to Burnaby?**

   a. About 10 miles
   b. About 5 miles
   c. About 15 miles
   d. About 20 miles

**18. How is the Village Hall from Victoria?**

   a. About 10 miles
   b. About 5 miles
   c. About 15 miles
   d. About 20 miles

**Questions 19 - 22 refer to the following passage.**

**Chocolate Chip Cookies**

3/4 cup sugar
3/4 cup packed brown sugar
1 cup butter, softened
2 large eggs, beaten
1 teaspoon vanilla extract
2 1/4 cups all-purpose flour
1 teaspoon baking soda
3/4 teaspoon salt
2 cups semisweet chocolate chips
If desired, 1 cup chopped pecans, or chopped walnuts.
Preheat oven to 375 degrees.

Mix sugar, brown sugar, butter, vanilla and eggs in a large bowl. Stir in flour, baking soda, and salt. The dough will be very stiff.

Stir in chocolate chips by hand with a sturdy wooden spoon. Add the pecans, or other nuts, if desired. Stir until the chocolate chips and nuts are evenly dispersed.

Drop dough by rounded tablespoonfuls 2 inches apart onto a cookie sheet.

Bake 8 to 10 minutes, or, until light brown. Cookies may look underdone, but they will finish cooking after you take them out of the oven.

**19. What is the correct order for adding these ingredients?**

   a. Brown sugar, baking soda, chocolate chips
   b. Baking soda, brown sugar, chocolate chips
   c. Chocolate chips, baking soda, brown sugar
   d. Baking soda, chocolate chips, brown sugar

**20. What does sturdy mean?**

   a. Long
   b. Strong
   c. Short
   d. Wide

**21. What does disperse mean?**

    a. Scatter

    b. To form a ball

    c. To stir

    d. To beat

**22. When can you stop stirring the nuts?**

    a. When the cookies are cooked.

    b. When the nuts are evenly distributed.

    c. When the nuts are added.

    d. After the chocolate chips are added.

**Questions 23 - 26 refer to the following passage.**

**Passage 5 - Winged Victory of Samothrace: the Statue of the Gods**

Students who read about the "Winged Victory of Samothrace" probably won't be able to visualize the statue. However, almost anyone who knows a little about statues will recognize it when they see it: it is the statue of a winged woman who does not have arms or a head. Even the most famous pieces of art may be recognized by sight but not by name.

This iconic statue is of the Greek goddess Nike, who represented victory and was called Victoria by the Romans. The statue is sometimes called the "Nike of Samothrace." She was often displayed in Greek art as driving a chariot, and her speed or efficiency with the chariot may be what her wings symbolize. It is said that the statue was created around 200 BCE to celebrate a battle that was won at sea. Archaeologists and art historians believe the statue originally may have been part of a temple or other building, even one of the most important temples, Megaloi Theoi, just as many statues were used during that time.

"Winged Victory" does indeed appear to have had arms and a head when it was originally created, and it is unclear why they were removed or lost. Indeed, they have never been discovered, even with all the excavation that has taken place. Many speculate that one of her arms was raised and put to her mouth, as though she was shouting or calling out, which is consistent with the idea of her as a war figure. If the missing pieces were ever to be found, they might give Greek and art historians more of an idea of what Nike represented or how the statue was used. Learning about pieces of art through details like these can help students remember time frames or locations, as well as learn about the people who occupied them.

**23. Why does the title says the statue is "of the Gods?"**

   a. The statue is very beautiful and even a god would find it beautiful

   b. The statue is of a Greek goddess, and gods were of primary importance to the Greek

   c. Nike lead the gods into war

   d. The statues were used at the temple of the gods and so it belonged to them

**24. The third paragraph states that**

   a. the statue is related to war and was probably broken apart by foreign soldiers

   b. the arms and head of the statue cannot be found because all the excavation has taken place

   c. speculations have been made about what the entire statue looked like and what it symbolized

   d. the statue has no arms or head because the sculptor lost them

**25. The author's main purpose in writing this passage is to**

   a. demonstrate that art and culture are related and one can teach us about the other

   b. persuade readers to become archaeologists and find the missing pieces of the statue

   c. teach readers about the Greek goddess Nike

   d. to teach readers the name of a statue they probably recognize

**26. The author specifies the indirect audience as "students" because**

   a. it is probably a student who is taking this test

   b. most young people don't know much about art yet and most young people are students

   c. students read more than people who are not students

   d. the passage is based on a discussion of what we can learn about culture from art

**Questions 27 - 29 refer to the following passage.**

**Lowest Price Guarantee**

**Get it for less. Guaranteed!**

ABC Electric will beat any advertised price by 10% of the difference.

1) If you find a lower advertised price, we will beat it by 10% of the difference.

2) If you find a lower advertised price within 30 days* of your purchase we will beat it by 10% of the difference.

3) If our own price is reduced within 30 days* of your purchase, bring in your receipt and we will refund the difference.

*14 days for computers, monitors, printers, laptops, tablets, cellular & wireless devices, home security products, projectors, camcorders, digital cameras, radar detectors, portable DVD players, DJ and pro-audio equipment, and air conditioners.

**27. I bought a radar detector 15 days ago and saw an ad for the same model only cheaper. Can I get 10% of the difference refunded?**

    a. Yes. Since it is less than 30 days, you can get 10% of the difference refunded.

    b. No. Since it is more than 14 days, you cannot get 10% of the difference re-funded.

    c. It depends on the cashier.

    d. Yes. You can get the difference refunded.

**28. I bought a flat-screen TV for $500 10 days ago and found an advertisement for the same TV, at another store, on sale for $400. How much will ABC refund under this guarantee?**

    a. $100
    b. $110
    c. $10
    d. $400

**29. What is the purpose of this passage?**

    a. To inform
    b. To educate
    c. To persuade
    d. To entertain

**Questions 30 - 33 refer to the following passage.**

**Passage 6 - What Is Mardi Gras?**

Mardi Gras is fast becoming one of the South's most famous and most celebrated holidays. The word Mardi Gras comes from the French and the literal translation is "Fat Tuesday." The holiday has also been called Shrove Tuesday, due to its associations with Lent. The purpose of Mardi Gras is to celebrate and enjoy before the Lenten season of fasting and repentance begins.

What originated by the French Explorers in New Orleans, Louisiana in the 17th century is now celebrated all over the world. Panama, Italy, Belgium and Brazil all host large scale Mardi Gras celebrations, and many smaller cities and towns celebrate this fun loving Tuesday as well. Usually held in February or early March, Mardi Gras is a day of extravagance, a day for people to eat, drink and be merry, to wear costumes, masks and to dance to jazz music.
The French explorers on the Mississippi River would be in shock today if they saw the opulence of the parades and floats that grace the New Orleans streets during Mardi Gras these days. Parades in New Orleans are divided by organizations. These are more commonly known as Krewes.

Being a member of a Krewe is quite a task because Krewes are responsible for overseeing the parades. Each Krewe's parade is ruled by a Mardi Gras "King and Queen." The role of the King and Queen is to "bestow" gifts on their adoring fans as the floats ride along the street. They throw doubloons, which is fake money and usually colored green, purple and gold, which are the colors of Mardi Gras. Beads in those color shades are also thrown and cups are thrown as well. Beads are by far the most popular souvenir of any Mardi Gras parade, with each spectator attempting to gather as many as possible.

**30. The purpose of Mardi Gras is to**

    a. Repent for a month.

    b. Celebrate in extravagant ways.

    c. Be a member of a Krewe.

    d. Explore the Mississippi.

**31. From reading the passage we can infer that "Kings and Queens,"**

    a. Have to be members of a Krewe.

    b. Have to be French.

    c. Have to know how to speak French.

    d. Have to give away their own money.

**32. Which group of people began to hold Mardi Gras celebrations?**

a. Settlers from Italy

b. Members of Krewes

c. French explorers

d. Belgium explorers

**33. In the context of the passage, what does spectator mean?**

a. Someone who participates actively

b. Someone who watches the parade's action

c. Someone on the parade floats

d. Someone who does not celebrate Mardi Gras

## Verbal Ability Part II – Vocabulary

**34. Choose the adjective that means shocking, terrible or wicked.**

a. Pleasantries

b. Heinous

c. Shrewd

d. Provencal

**35. Choose the noun that means a person or thing that tells or announces the coming of someone or something.**

a. Harbinger

b. Evasion

c. Bleak

d. Craven

**36. Choose a word that means the same as the underlined word.**

**He wasn't especially generous. All the servings were very <u>judicious</u>.**

    a. Abundant

    b. Careful

    c. Extravagant

    d. Careless

**37. Fill in the blank.**

**Because of the growing use of _____ as a fuel, corn production has greatly increased.**

    a. Alcohol

    b. Ethanol

    c. Natural gas

    d. Oil

**38. Fill in the blank.**

**In heavily industrialized areas, the pollution of the air causes many to develop _____ diseases.**

    a. Respiratory

    b. Cardiac

    c. Alimentary

    d. Circulatory

**39. Choose the best definition of inherent.**

    a. To receive money in a will

    b. An essential part of

    c. To receive money from a will

    d. None of the above

**40. Choose the best definition of vapid.**

    a. adj. Tasteless or bland

    b. v. To inflict, as a revenge or punishment

    c. v. To convert into gas

    d. v. To go up in smoke

**41. Choose the best definition of waif.**

    a. n. A sick and hungry child

    b. n. An orphan staying in a foster home

    c. n. Homeless child or stray

    d. n. A type of French bread eaten with cheese

**42. Choose the adjective that means similar or identical.**

    a. Soluble

    b. Assembly

    c. Conclave

    d. Homologous

**43. Choose a word with the same meaning as the underlined word.**

**We used that operating system 20 years ago, now it is <u>obsolete</u>.**

    a. Functional

    b. Disused

    c. Obese

    d. None of the Above

**44. Choose the word with the same meaning as the underlined word**

**His bad manners really <u>rankle</u> me.**

    a. Annoy

    b. Obsolete

    c. Enliven

    d. None of the above

**45. Fill in the blank.**

**Because hydroelectric power is a _____ source of energy, its use is excellent for the environment.**

    a. Significant

    b. Disposable

    c. Renewable

    d. Reusable

**46. Choose the best definition of torpid.**

    a. Fast

    b. Rapid

    c. Sluggish

    d. Violent

**47. Choose the best definition of gregarious.**

    a. Sociable

    b. Introverted

    c. Large

    d. Solitary

**48. Choose the best definition of mutation.**

    a. v. To utter with a loud and vehement voice

    b. n. Change or alteration

    c. n. An act or exercise of will

    d. v. To cause to be one

**49. Choose the best definition of lithe.**

    a. adj. Small in size

    b. adj. Artificial

    c. adj. Flexible or plaint

    d. adj. Fake

**50. Choose the best definition of resent.**

    a. adj. To express displeasure or indignation

    b. v. To cause to be one

    c. adj. Clumsy

    d. adj. Strong feelings of love

**51. Choose the adjective that means irrelevant not having substance or matter.**

    a. Immaterial

    b. Prohibition

    c. Prediction

    d. Brokerage

**52. Choose the adjective that means perfect, no faults or errors.**

    a. Impeccable

    b. Formidable

    c. Genteel

    d. Disputation

**53. Choose the best definition of pudgy.**

   a. v. To draw general inferences
   b. Adj. fat, plump and overweight
   c. n. Permanence
   d. adj. Spoilt or bad condition

**54. Choose the best definition of alloy.**

   a. To mix with something superior
   b. To mix
   c. To mix with something inferior
   d. To purify

**55. Fill in the blank.**

The process required the use of highly _____ liquids, so fire extinguishers were everywhere in the factory.

   a. Erratic
   b. Combustible
   c. Stable
   d. Neutral

**56. Choose the best definition for the underlined word.**

We don't want to hear the whole thing. Just the <u>salient</u> facts please.

   a. Irrelevant
   b. Erroneous
   c. Relevant
   d. Trivial

**57. Choose the best definition for the underlined word.**

I don't know why he is being so nice. I am sure he has an <u>ulterior</u> motive.

   a. Inferior
   b. Additional
   c. Simplistic
   d. Unfortunate

**58. Choose the noun that means ruling council of a military government.**

   a. Retribution
   b. Counsel
   c. Virago
   d. Junta

**59. Choose a noun that means someone who takes more time than necessary.**

   a. Manager
   b. Haggard
   c. Laggard
   d. Expound

**60. Choose an adjective that means lacking enthusiasm, strength or energy.**

   a. Hapless
   b. Languid
   c. Ubiquitous
   d. Promiscuous

## Section II – Math

**1.** It is known that $x^2 + 4x = 5$. Then x can be

    a. 0
    b. -5
    c. 1
    d. Either (b) or (c)

**2.** $(a + b)2 = 4ab$. What is necessarily correct?

    a. a > b
    b. a < b
    c. a = b
    d. None of the Above

**3.** The sum of the digits of a 2-digit number is 12. If we switch the digits, the resulting number will be greater than the initial one by 36. Find the initial number.

    a. 39
    b. 48
    c. 57
    d. 75

**4.** In a class of 83 students, 72 are present. What percent of student is absent?

    a. 12
    b. 13
    c. 14
    d. 15

**5.** Kate's father is 32 years older than Kate is. In 5 years, he will be five times older. How old is Kate?

    a. 2
    b. 3
    c. 5
    d. 6

**6.** If Lynn can type a page in p minutes, what portion of the page can she do in 5 minutes?

    a. 5/p
    b. p - 5
    c. p + 5
    d. p/5

**7.** Find the mean of these set of numbers – 2.5, 10.2, 4.5, 1.25, 7.05, 20.8

    a. 7.6
    b. 45.6
    c. 7
    d. 1.25

**8.** If Sally can paint a house in 4 hours, and John can paint the same house in 6 hours, how long will it take for both of them to paint the house together?

    a. 2 hours and 24 minutes
    b. 3 hours and 12 minutes
    c. 3 hours and 44 minutes
    d. 4 hours and 10 minutes

**9.** A bullet weighing 350g is shot towards a target at a velocity of 250m/s. Calculate the momentum of the bullet?

    a. 1.4 kg x m/s towards target
    b. 87.5 kg x m/s towards target
    c. 87500 kg x m/s towards target
    d. 8.75 kg x m/s towards target

**10. Using the quadratic formula, solve the quadratic equation: $x^2 - 9x + 14 = 0$**

   a. 2 and 7

   b. -2 and 7

   c. -7 and -2

   d. -7 and 2

**11. Employees of a discount appliance store receive an additional 20% off the lowest price on any item. If an employee purchases a dishwasher during a 15% off sale, how much will he pay if the dishwasher originally cost $450?**

   a. $280.90

   b. $287.00

   c. $292.50

   d. $306.00

**12. The sale price of a car is $12,590, which is 20% off the original price. What is the original price?**

   a. $14,310.40

   b. $14,990.90

   c. $15,108.00

   d. $15,737.50

**13. A goat eats 214 kg. of hay in 60 days, while a cow eats the same amount in 15 days. How long will it take them to eat this hay together?**

   a. 37.5

   b. 75

   c. 12

   d. 15

**14. Express 125% as a decimal.**

   a. .125

   b. 12.5

   c. 1.25

   d. 125

**15. What are the prime factors of 125?**

   a. 5 x 25

   b. 5 x 5 x 5

   d. All of the above

   d. None of the above

**16. Solve for x: 30 is 40% of x**

   a. 60

   b. 90

   c. 85

   d. 75

**17. Which of these object has greater momentum, a 2kg truck moving east at 3.5m/s or a 4.3kg truck moving south at 1.5m/s?**

   a. The first truck at 7 kg x m/s moving east

   b. The second truck at 7.45 kg x m/s due south

   c. The first truck at 6.45 kg x m/s due east

   d. The second truck at 7 kg x m/s due south

**18. 12 ½% of x is equal to 50. Solve for x.**

   a. 300

   b. 400

   c. 450

   d. 350

**19. Express 24/56 as a reduced common fraction.**

   a. 4/9

   b. 4/11

   c. 3/7

   d. 3/8

**20. What are the prime factors of 132?**

    a. 4 x 3 x 11
    b. 2 x 2 x 2 x 3 x 11
    c. 2 x 6 x 11
    d. 2 x 2 x 3 x 11

**21. Express 87% as a decimal.**

    a. .087
    b. 8.7
    c. .87
    d. 87

**22. 60 is 75% of x. Solve for x.**

    a. 80
    b. 90
    c. 75
    d. 70

**23. Find the median of these set of test scores taken from a class of students – 90, 80, 77, 86, 50, 91, 73, 66, 69, 45, 43, 65, 75**

    a. 13
    b. 73
    c. 9
    d. 706

**24. 4.7 + .9 + .01 =**

    a. 5.5
    b. 6.51
    c. 5.61
    d. 5.7

**25. .87 - .48 =**

    a. .39
    b. .49
    c. .41
    d. .37

**26. The physician ordered 100 mg Ibuprofen/kg of body weight; on hand is 230 mg/tablet. The child weighs 50 lb. How many tablets will you give?**

    a. 10 tablets
    b. 5 tablets
    c. 1 tablet
    d. 12 tablets

**27. Find the mode from these numbers – 7,2,3,9,6,5,1,4,8**

    a. 1
    b. 5
    c. 9
    d. None of the above

**28. Simplify $4^3$**

    a. 20
    b. 32
    c. 64
    d. 108

**29. The physician ordered 5 mL of Capacitate; 15 mL/tsp is on hand. How many teaspoons will you give?**

    a. 0.05 tsp
    b. 0.03 tsp
    c. 0.5 tsp
    d. 0.3 tsp

**30.** Using the quadratic formula, solve the quadratic equation: $x - 31/x = 0$

   a. $-\sqrt{13}$ and $\sqrt{13}$
   b. $-\sqrt{31}$ and $\sqrt{31}$
   c. $-\sqrt{31}$ and $2\sqrt{31}$
   d. $-\sqrt{3}$ and $\sqrt{3}$

**31.** The manager of a weaving factory estimates that if 10 machines run on 100% efficiency for 8 hours, they will produce 1450 meters of cloth. However, due to some technical problems, 4 machines run of 95% efficiency and the remaining 6 at 90% efficiency. How many meters of cloth can these machines will produce in 8 hours?

   a. 1334 meters
   b. 1310 meters
   c. 1300 meters
   d. 1285 meters

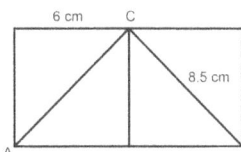

Note: figure not drawn to scale

**32.** Assuming the 2 quadrangles in the figure are identical rectangles, what is the perimeter of △ABC in the above shape?

   a. 25.5 cm
   b. 27 cm
   c. 30 cm
   d. 29 cm

**33.** Solve for x if, $10^2 \times 100^2 = 1000^x$

   a. $x = 2$
   b. $x = 3$
   c. $x = -2$
   d. $x = 0$

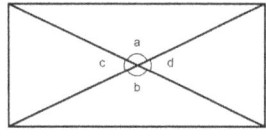

**34.** What is the sum of angles a, b, c and d in the rectangle above?

   a. 180°
   b. 360°
   c. 90°
   d. 120°

**35.** Find the mode from these test results – 2, 4, 2, 6, 4, 9, 6, 7, 2, 9, 7, 6, 4, 10, 10, 2, 6, 7, 9

   a. 2 and 9
   b. 2
   c. 2 and 6
   d. 2 and 7

**36.** Convert from scientific notation: $5.63 \times 10^6$

   a. 5,630,000
   b. 563,000
   c. 5630
   d. 0.000005.630

**37. 30 mg is the same mass as:**

a. 0.0003 kg.
b. 0.03 grams
c. 300 decigrams
d. 0.3 grams

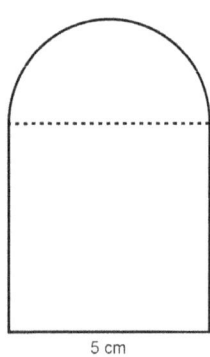

Note: figure not drawn to scale

**38. What is the perimeter of the above shape?**

a. 17.5 π cm
b. 20 π cm
c. 15 π cm
d. 25 π cm

**39. 0.101 mm. =**

a. .0101 cm
b. 1.01 cm
c. 0.00101 cm
d. 10.10 cm

**40. Using the factoring method, solve the quadratic equation: $2x^2 - 3x = 0$**

a. 0 and 1.5
b. 1.5 and 2
c. 2 and 2.5
d. 0 and 2

**41. How much water can be stored in a cylindrical container 5 meters in diameter and 12 meters high?**

a. 223.65 m$^3$
b. 235.65 m$^3$
c. 240.65 m$^3$
d. 252.65 m$^3$

**42. Convert 0.045 to scientific notation.**

a. $4.5 \times 10^{-2}$
b. $4.5 \times 10^{2}$
c. $4.05 \times 10^{-2}$
d. $4.5 \times 10^{-3}$

43.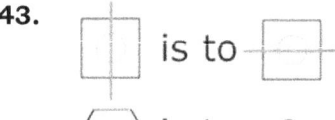

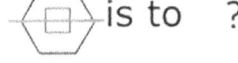

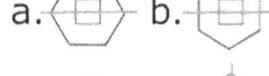

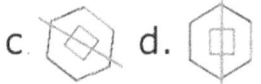

44.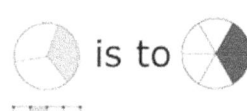

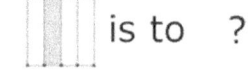

**45.**

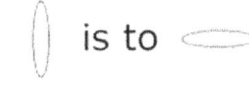

| is to ⬯

△ is to ?

a. ▷ b. ◇

c. ◇ d. △

**46.** ⬚ is to ⬡

⬚ is to ?

a. ⬠ b. ◯

c. ◻ d. △

**47. Factor the polynomial 9x² - 6x + 12.**

 a. $3(x^2 - 2x + 9)$
 b. $3(3x^2 - 3x + 4)$
 c. $9(x^2 - 3x + 3)$
 d. $3(3x^2 - 2x + 4)$

**48. 389 + 454 =**

 a. 853
 b. 833
 c. 843
 d. 863

**49. 9,177 + 7,204 =**

 a. 16,4712
 b. 16,371
 c. 16,381
 d. 15,412

**50. 2,199 + 5,832 =**

 a. 8,331
 b. 8,041
 c. 8,141
 d. 8,031

## Section III – Science

**1. A soccer ball is kicked and travels at a velocity of 12 m/sec. After 60 seconds, it comes to a stop. What is the acceleration?**

   a. -0.2 m/sec$^2$
   b. 0.2 m/sec$^2$
   c. 1 m/sec$^2$
   d. 0.5 m/sec$^2$

**2. A molecule of water contains hydrogen and oxygen in a 1:8 ratio by mass. This is a statement of**

   a. The law of multiple proportions
   b. The law of conservation of mass
   c. The law of conservation of energy
   d. The law of constant composition

**3. Electrons play a critical role in**

   a. Electricity
   b. Magnetism
   c. Thermal conductivity
   d. All of the above

**4. An idea concerning a phenomena and possible explanations for that phenomena is a/an**

   a. Theory.
   b. Experiment.
   c. Inference.
   d. Hypothesis.

**5. Define chromosomes.**

   a. Structures in a cell nucleus that carry genetic material.
   b. Consist of thousands of DNA strands.
   c. Total 46 in a normal human cell.
   d. All of the above

**6. A base is**

    a. A compound that reacts with an acid to form a salt.

    b. A molecule or ion that captures hydrogen ions.

    c. A molecule or ion that donates an electron pair to form a chemical bond.

    d. All of the above are true

**7. Which disease of the circulatory system is one of the most frequent causes of death in North America?**

    a. The cold

    b. Pneumonia

    c. Arthritis

    d. Heart disease

**8. How fast can a person walk if they travel 1000 m in 20 minutes?**

    a. 25 meters

    b. 50 meters

    c. 100 meters

    d. None of the above

**9. A substance containing atoms of more than one element in a definite ratio is called a(n)**

    a. Compound

    b. Element

    c. Mixture

    d. Molecule

**10. Which of the following describes a plasma membrane?**

    a. Lipids with embedded proteins

    b. An outer lipid layer and an inner lipid layer

    c. Proteins embedded in lipid bilayer

    d. Altering protein and lipid layers

**11. Protein biosynthesis is defined as**

   a. The addition of protein to foods that lack it.
   b. Ribosomes synthesizing proteins in the endoplasmic reticulum.
   c. The process of proteasomes degrading cytoplasm.
   d. Proteins "flowing" through the ER into the plasma membrane.

**12. When we speak of separating organelles through centrifugation, we're speaking of**

   a. Cell fractionation
   b. Flow cytometry
   c. Immunoprecipation
   d. Detergents

**13. What is the difference between Strong Nuclear Force and Weak Nuclear Force?**

   a. The Strong Nuclear Force is an attractive force that binds protons and neutrons and maintains the structure of the nucleus, and the Weak Nuclear Force is responsible for the radioactive beta decay and other subatomic reactions.

   b. The Strong Nuclear Force is responsible for the radioactive beta decay and other subatomic reactions, and the Weak Nuclear Force is an attractive force that binds protons and neutrons and maintains the structure of the nucleus.

   c. The Weak Nuclear Force is feeble and the Strong Nuclear Force is robust.

   d. The Strong Nuclear Force is a negative force that releases protons and neutrons and threatens the structure of the nucleus, and the Weak Nuclear Force is an attractive force that binds protons and neutrons and maintains the structure of the nucleus.

**14. 1000 N force is applied to a concrete block that weights 500 pounds. How fast will this force accelerate the block?**

   a. $1 \text{ m/sec}^2$
   b. $2 \text{ m/sec}^2$
   c. $3 \text{ m/sec}^2$
   d. $5 \text{ m/sec}^2$

**15. What type of research deals with the quality, type or components of a group, substance, or mixture.**

   a. Quantitative
   b. Dependent
   c. Scientific
   d. Qualitative

**16. When a measurement is recorded, it includes the _____ _____, which are all the digits that are certain plus one uncertain digit.**

   a. Major figures
   b. Significant figures
   c. Relative figures
   d. Relevant figures

**17. The equation E = mc² is based on the _____, and states that _____ equals \_\_\_\_\_ times the _____².**

   a. The equation $E = mc^2$ is based on the 2nd Law of Thermodynamics, and states that Mass equals Energy times (the Velocity of light)².
   b. The equation $E = mc^2$ is based on the Law of Conservation of Mass and Energy, and states that Energy equals Mass times (the Velocity of light)².
   c. The equation $E = mc^2$ is based on the 1st Law of Thermodynamics, and states that Mass equals Energy times (the Velocity of sound)².
   d. The equation $E = mc^2$ is based on the Law of Conservation of Mass and Energy, and states that the Velocity of light equals Energy times (the Mass)².

**18. Describe a pH indicator.**

   a. A pH indicator measures hydrogen ions in a solution and show pH on a color scale.
   b. A pH indicator measures oxygen ions in a solution and show pH on a color scale.
   c. A pH indicator many different types of ions in a solution and shows pH on a color scale
   d. None of the above

**19. All acids turn blue litmus paper**

   a. Blue
   b. Red
   c. Green
   d. White

20. **What type of bonds involve a complete sharing of electrons and occurs most commonly between atoms that have partially filled outer shells or energy levels?**

   a. Covalent
   b. Ionic
   c. Hydrogen
   d. Proportional

21. **What can accept a hydrogen ion and can react with fats to form soap?**

   a. Acid
   b. Salt
   c. Base
   d. Foundation

22. **Which, if any, of the following statements are true?**

   a. Water boils at about 100 °C (212 °F) at standard atmospheric pressure.
   b. The boiling point is the temperature at which the vapor pressure is higher than the atmospheric pressure around the water.
   c. Water boils at a higher temperature in areas of lower pressure.
   d. All of the above statements are true.

23. **Which gene, whose presence as a single copy, controls the expression of a trait?**

   a. Principal gene
   b. Latent gene
   c. Recessive gene
   d. Dominant gene

24. **What is the mathematical function that gives the amplitude of a wave as a function of position (and sometimes, as a function of time and/or electron spin)?**

   a. Wavelength
   b. Frequency
   c. Wavenumber
   d. Wavefunction

**25. Which of the following is not a habitat where bacteria commonly grow?**

   a. Soil
   b. The vacuum of space
   c. Radioactive waste
   d. Deep in the earth's crust

**26. Within taxonomy, plants and animals are considered two basic**

   a. Families
   b. Kingdoms
   c. Domains
   d. Genus

**27. How much force is needed to accelerate a car that weights 200 kg to 5 m/s²?**

   a. 2000 N
   b. 4000 N
   c. 6000 N
   d. 8000 N

**28. What is a chemical involved in, but not changed by, a chemical reaction by which chemical bonds are weakened and reactions accelerated.**

   a. A propellant
   b. A reagent
   c. A catalyst
   d. None of the above

**29. Organisms grouped into the _____ Kingdom include all unicellular organisms lacking a definite cellular arrangement such as _____ and _____.**

   a. Fungi, bacteria, algae
   b. Protista, bacteria, amphibian
   c. Protista, bacteria, algae
   d. Plantae, bacteria, algae

**30. Which of these statements about metals are true?**

a. A metal is a substance that conducts heat and electricity.

b. A metal is shiny and reflects many colors of light, and can be hammered into sheets or drawn into wire.

c. All these statements are true.

d. About 80% of the known chemical elements are metals.

**31. What type of bond does a reaction of elements with low electronegativity (almost empty outer shells) with elements with high electronegativity (mostly full outer shells) create?**

a. Hydrogen

b. Covalent

c. Ionic

d. Nuclear

**32. Which of the following is not an infectious bacterial disease?**

a. Cholera

b. Anthrax

c. Leprosy

d. AIDS

**33. Define a biological class.**

a. A collection of similar or like living entities.

b. Two or more animals in a group, all having the same parent.

c. All animals sharing the same living environment.

d. All plant life that share the same physical properties.

**34. Which, if any, of the following statements about prokaryotic cells is false?**

a. Prokaryotic cells include such organisms as E. coli and Streptococcus.

b. Prokaryotic cells lack internal membranes and organelles.

c. Prokaryotic cells break down food using cellular respiration and fermentation.

d. All of these statements are true.

**35. 1000 N force is applied to a concrete block that weights 500 pounds. How fast will this force accelerate the block?**

    a. -2 m/sec²

    b. 2 m/sec²

    c. 4 m/sec²

    d. 5 m/sec²

**36. What is the process of converting observed phenomena into data is called?**

    a. Calculation

    b. Measurement

    c. Valuation

    d. Estimation

**37. What law states that when two elements combine with to form more than one compound, the weights of one element that combine with a fixed weight of the other are in a ratio of small whole numbers?**

    a. The Law of Multiple Proportions

    b. The Law of Definite Proportions

    c. The Law of the Conservation of Energy

    d. The Law of Averages

**38. What word describes the wide diversity of sizes and shapes found in bacteria?**

    a. Morphologies

    b. Cosmologies

    c. Proteins

    d. Spirilla

**39. The mass number of an atom is**

    a. The total number of particles that make it up.

    b. The total weight of an atom.

    c. The total mass of an atom.

    d. None of the above.

**40. Which of these statements about mechanical energy is/are true?**

a. Mechanical energy is the energy an object possesses due to its motion or due to its position.

b. Mechanical energy can be either kinetic energy (energy of motion) or potential energy (stored energy of position).

c. Objects have mechanical energy if they are in motion.

d. All of the above.

**41. What three processes are involved in cell division of Eukaryotic cells?**

a. Meiosis, mitosis, and interphase

b. Meiosis, mitosis, and interphase

c. Mitosis, kinematisis, and interphase

d. Mitosis, cytokinesis, and interphase

**42. The _____ _____ of an element equals the number of protons in an atomic nucleus, and, along with the element symbol is one of two alternate ways to label an element.**

a. Atomic unit

b. Atomic number

c. Atomic orbital

d. Nuclear number

**43. Which of the following statements, if any, are correct?**

a. pH is a measure of effective concentration of hydrogen ions in a solution, and is approximately related to the molarity of H+ by pH = - log [H+]

b. pH is a measure of effective concentration of oxygen ions in a solution, and is approximately related to the molarity of O+ by pH = - log [O+]

c. pH is a measure of effective concentration of hydrogen atoms in a solution, and is approximately related to the polarity of H+ by pH = - log [H+]

d. Acidity is a measure of effective concentration of hydrogen ions in a solution, and is approximately related to the molarity of H+ by pH = - log [H+]

**44. What chain of nucleotides plays an important role in the creation of new proteins?**

    a. Deoxyribonucleic acid (DNA) is a chain of nucleotides that plays an important role in the creation of new proteins.

    b. Ribonucleic acid (RNA) is a chain of nucleotides that plays an important role in the creation of new proteins.

    c. There are no chains of nucleotides that play a role in the creation of proteins.

    d. None of the above.

**45. How much force is needed to accelerate a car that weights 200 kg to 5 m/s$^2$?**

    a. 40 N

    b. 200 N

    c. 1000 N

    d. 1500 N

**46. What law states that every chemical compound contains fixed and constant proportions (by weight) of its constituent elements?**

    a. The Law of Multiple Proportions

    b. The Law of the Preservation of Matter

    c. The Law of the Conservation of Energy

    d. The Law of Definite Proportions

**47. Four factors that affect rates of reaction are**

    a. Barometric pressure, particle size, concentration, and the presence of a facilitator.

    b. Temperature, particle size, concentration, and the presence of a catalyst.

    c. Temperature, container material, elevation, and the presence of instability.

    d. Volatility, particle size, concentration, and the presence of a catalyst.

**48. What is the term used for bacterial species which are spherical in shape?**

    a. Bacilli

    b. Spirilla

    c. Cocci

    d. Spirochaetes

**49. A practical test designed with the intention that its results will be relevant to a particular theory or set of theories is a/an _____.**

   a. Experiment
   b. Practicum
   c. Theory
   d. Design

**50. If 3 moles of sugar is dissolved to form 2 liters of a solution, calculate the molarity of the solution.**

   a. 1 M solution
   b. 1.5 M solution
   c. 2 M solution
   d. 2.5 M solution

**51. Electricity is a general term encompassing a variety of phenomena resulting from the presence and flow of electric charge. Which of the following statements about electricity is/are true?**

   a. Electrically charged matter is influenced by, and produces, electromagnetic fields.
   b. Electric current is a movement or flow of electrically charged particles.
   c. Electric potential is a fundamental interaction between the magnetic field and the presence and motion of an electric charge.
   d. All of the statements are true.

**52. Strong chemical bonds include**

   a. Dipole - dipole interactions
   b. Hydrogen bonding
   c. Covalent or ionic bonds
   d. None of the above

**53. A javelin is thrown into a field at 18 m/s. if the Javelin weighs 1.5 kg, what is the momentum?**

   a. 1.2 kg x m/s into the field
   b. 12 kg x m/s into the field
   c. 27 kg x m/s into the field
   d. 2.7 kg x m/s into the field

**54. Which of these object has greater momentum, a 2 kg truck moving east at 3.5 m/s or a 4.3 kg truck moving south at 1.5 m/s?**

   a. The first truck at 7 kg x m/s moving east

   b. The second truck at 7.45 kg x m/s due south

   c. The first truck at 6.45 kg x m/s due east

   d. The second truck at 7 kg x m/s due south

**55. What is the measure of an experiment's ability to yield the same or compatible results in different clinical experiments or statistical trials?**

   a. Variability

   b. Validity

   c. Control measure

   d. Reliability

**56. Genes control heredity in man and other organisms. This gene is**

   a. a segment of RNA or DNA.

   b. a bead like structure on the chromosomes.

   c. a protein molecule.

   d. a segment of RNA.

**57. One factor that affects rates of reaction is concentration. Which of these statements about concentration is/are correct?**

   a. A higher concentration of reactants causes more effective collisions per unit time, leading to an increased reaction rate.

   b. A lower concentration of reactants causes more effective collisions per unit time, leading to an increased reaction rate.

   c. A higher concentration of reactants causes more effective collisions per unit time, leading to a decreased reaction rate.

   d. A higher concentration of reactants causes less effective collisions per unit time, leading to an increased reaction rate.

**58. Describe each chemical element in the periodic table.**

   a. Each chemical element has a unique atomic number representing the number of electrons in its nucleus.

   b. Each chemical element has a varying atomic number depending on the number of protons in its nucleus.

   c. Each chemical element has a unique atomic number representing the number of protons in its nucleus.

   d. None of the above.

**59. Which of the following statements about nonmetals are true?**

a. A nonmetal is a substance that conducts heat and electricity poorly.

b. Most known chemical elements are nonmetals.

c. A nonmetal is brittle or waxy or gaseous.

d. All of the statements are true.

**60. The molarity of 5 liters of a salt solution is 0.5 M of salt solution. Calculate the moles of salt in the solution.**

a. 2 Moles

b. 2.5 Moles

c. 2.75 Moles

d. 3 Moles

**61. A solution with a pH value of less than 7 is**

a. Acid solution

b. Base solution

c. Neutral pH solution

d. None of the above

**62. What is the distance between adjacent peaks (or adjacent troughs) on a wave?**

a. Frequency

b. Wavenumber

c. Wave oscillation

d. Wavelength

**63. An object that weighs 500 g is rolling along the road at 3.5 m/s. What is the momentum of the object?**

a. 124.9 kg x m/s along road

b. 17. 50 kg x m/s along road

c. 1750 kg x m/s along road

d. 1.75 kg x m/s along road

**64. Is a catalyst changed by a reaction?**

   a. Yes

   b. No

   c. It may be changed depending on the other chemicals

**65. The _____ is the prediction that an observed difference is due to chance alone and not due to a systematic cause; this hypothesis is tested by statistical analysis, and either accepted or rejected.**

   a. Null hypothesis

   b. Hypothesis

   c. Control

   d. Variable

**66. In science, industry, and statistics, the _____ of a measurement system is the degree of closeness of measurements of a quantity to its actual (true) value.**

   a. Mistake

   b. Uncertainty

   c. Accuracy

   d. Error

**67. The horizontal rows of the periodic table are known as**

   a. Groups

   b. Periods

   c. Series

   d. Columns

**68. Which, if any, of these statements about solubility are correct?**

   a. The solubility of a substance is its concentration in a saturated solution.

   b. Substances with solubilities much less than 1 g/100 mL of solvent are usually considered insoluble.

   c. A saturated solution is one which does not dissolve any more solute.

   d. All of these statements are correct.

**69. Describe a valence shell.**

a. Is the shell corresponding to the highest value of principal quantum number in the atom.

b. The valence electrons in this shell are on average closer to the nucleus than other electrons.

c. They are rarely directly involved in chemical reaction.

d. None of the above are true.

**70. To calculate the Molarity of a solution when the solute is given in grams and the volume of the solution is given in milliliters, you must first**

a. Convert grams to moles, but leave the volume of solution in milliliters.

b. Convert volume of solution in milliliters to liters, but leave grams to moles.

c. Convert grams to moles, and convert volume of solution in milliliters to liters.

d. None of the above.

**71. What is the atomic number for Hydrogen?**

a. 11

b. 2

c. 1

d. 5

**72. The vertical columns of the periodic table are known as**

a. Series

b. Groups

c. Periods

d. Columns

**73. The ____ of a distribution is the difference between the maximum value and the minimum value.**

a. Distribution

b. Range

c. Mode

d. Median

**74. A cannon ball weighing 35 kg is shot from a cannon towards the east at 220m/s, calculate the momentum of the cannon ball.**

   a. 7500 kg m/s east
   b. 7700 kg m/s east
   c. 8000 kg m/s east
   d. 8500 kg m/s east

**75. Which, if any, of the following statements describing acids are correct?**

   a. An acid is a compound containing detachable hydrogen ions.
   b. An acid is a compound that can accept a pair of electrons from a base.
   c. A and B are correct
   d. None of the above

## Answer Key

**1. A**
Choice B is incorrect; the author did not express their opinion on the subject matter. Choice C is incorrect, the author was not trying to prove a point, nor is the author trying to persuade.

**2. C**
Choice C is correct; historians believe it was brutal and bloody. Choice A is incorrect; there is no consensus that the Crusades achieved great things. Choice B is incorrect; it did not stabilize the Holy Lands. Choice D is incorrect, some historians do believe this was the purpose but not all historians.

**3. D**
The feudal system led to infighting. Choice A is incorrect, it had the opposite effect. Choice B is incorrect, though this is a good answer, it is not the best answer. The Church asked for volunteers not the Feudal Lords. Choice C is incorrect, it did have an effect on the Crusades.

**4. A**
Saracen was a generic term for Muslims widely used in Europe during the later medieval era.

**5. B**
This warranty does not cover a product that you have tried to fix yourself. From paragraph two, "This limited warranty does not cover ... any unauthorized disassembly, repair, or modification. "

**6. C**
ABC Electric could either replace or repair the fan, provided the other conditions are met. ABC Electric has the option to repair or replace.

**7. B**
The warranty does not cover a stove damaged in a flood. From the passage, "This limited warranty does not cover any damage to the product from improper installation, accident, abuse, misuse, natural disaster, insufficient or excessive electrical supply, abnormal mechanical or environmental conditions."

A flood is an "abnormal environmental condition," and a natural disaster, so it is not covered.

**8. A**
A missing part is an example of defective workmanship. This is an error made in the manufacturing process. A defective part is not considered workmanship.

**9. D**
This question tests the reader's summarization skills. The other choices A, B, and C focus on portions of the second paragraph that are too narrow and do not relate to the specific portion of text in question. The complexity of the sentence may mislead students into selecting one of these answers, but rearranging or restating the sentence will lead the reader to the correct answer. In addition, choice A makes an assumption that may or may not be true about the intentions of the company, choice B focuses on one product rather than the idea of the products, and choice C makes an assumption about women that may or may not be true and is not supported by the text.

**10. B**
This question tests reader's attention to detail. If a reader selects A, he or she may have picked up on the use of the word "debate" and assumed, very logically, that the two are at odds because they are fighting; however, this is simply not supported in the text. Choice C also uses very specific quotes from the text, but it rearranges and gives them false meaning. The artists want to elevate their creations above the creations of other artists, thereby showing that they are "creative" and "innovative." Similarly, choice D takes phrases straight

from the text and rearranges and confuses them. The artists are described as wanting to be "creative, innovative, individual people," not the women.

**11. A**

This question tests reader's vocabulary and summarization skills. This phrase, used by the author, may seem flippant and dismissive if readers focus on the word "whatever" and misinterpret it as a popular, colloquial term. In this way, choices B and C may mislead the reader to selecting one of them by including the terms "unimportant" and "stupid," respectively. Choice D is a similar misreading, but doesn't make sense when the phrase is at the beginning of the passage and the entire passage is on media messages. Choice A is literally and contextually appropriate, and the reader can understand that the author would like to keep the introduction focused on the topic the passage is going to discuss.

**12. A**

This question tests a reader's inference skills. The extreme use of the word "all" in choice B suggests that every single advertising company are working to be approachable, and while this is not only unlikely, the text specifically states that "more" companies have done this, signifying that they have not all participated, even if it's a possibility that they may some day. The use of the limiting word "only" in choice C lends that answer similar problems; women are still buying from companies who do not care about this message, or those companies would not be in business, and the passage specifies that "many" women are worried about media messages, but not all. Readers may find choice D logical, especially if they are looking to make an inference, and while this may be a possibility, the passage does not suggest or discuss this happening. Choice A is correct based on specifically because of the relation between "still working" in the answer and "will hopefully" and the extensive discussion on companies struggles, which come only with progress, in the text.

**13. C**

This question tests the reader's summarization skills. The entire passage is leading up to the idea that the president of the US may not have had grounds to assert his Fourteen Points when other countries had lost so much. Choice A is pretty directly inferred by the text, but it does not adequately summarize what the entire passage is trying to communicate. Choice B may also be inferred by the passage when it says that the war is "imminent," but it does not represent the entire message, either. The passage does seem to be in praise of FDR, or at least in respect of him, but it does not in any way claim that he is the smartest president, nor does this represent the many other points included. Choice C is then the obvious answer, and most directly relates to the closing sentences which it rewords.

**14. C**

This question tests the reader's attention to detail. The passage does state that choices A and B are true, and while those statements are in proximity to the explanation for why the war started, they are not the reason given. Choice D is a mix up of words used in the passage, which says that the largest powers were in play but not that this fact somehow started the war. The passage does make a direct statement that a domino effect started the war, supporting choice C as the correct answer.

**15. A**

This question tests the reader's understanding of functions in writing. Throughout the passage, it states that leaders of other nations were hesitant to accept generous or peaceful terms because of the grievances of the war, and the great loss of life was chief among these. While the passage does touch on the devastation of deadly weapons (B), the use of this raw, emotional fact serves a much larger purpose, and the focus of the passage is not the weapons. While readers may indeed consider who lost the most soldiers (C) when, so many countries were involved and the inequalities of loss are mentioned in the passage, there is no discussion of this in the passage. Choice D is related to A, but choice A is more direct and relates more to the passage.

### 16. B
This question tests the reader's vocabulary skills. Choice A may seem appealing to readers because it is phonetically similar to "catalysed," but the two are not related in any other way. Choice C makes sense in context, but if plugged in to the sentence creates a redundancy that doesn't make sense. Choice D does also not make sense contextually, even if the reader may consider that funds were needed to create more weaponry, especially if it was advanced.

### 17. A
Victoria is about 5 miles from Burnaby.

### 18. B
The Village Hall is about 5 miles from Victoria.

### 19. A
The correct order of ingredients is brown sugar, baking soda and chocolate chips.

### 20. B
Sturdy: strong, solid in structure or person. In context, Stir in chocolate chips by hand with a *sturdy* wooden spoon.

### 21. A
Disperse: to scatter in different directions or break up. In context, Stir until the chocolate chips and nuts are evenly *dispersed*.

### 22. B
You can stop stirring the nuts when they are evenly distributed. From the passage, "Stir until the chocolate chips and nuts are evenly dispersed."

### 23. B
This question tests the reader's summarization skills. Choice A is a very broad statement that may or may not be true, and seems to be in context, but has nothing to do with the passage. The author does mention that the statue was probably used on a temple dedicated to the Greek gods (D), but in no way discusses or argues for the gods' attitude toward or claim on these temples or its faucets. Nike does indeed lead the gods into a war (the Titan war), as choice C suggests, but this is not mentioned by the passage and students who know this may be drawn to this answer but have not done a close enough analysis of the text that is actually in the passage. Choice B is appropriately expository, and connects the titular emphasis to the idea that the Greek gods are very important to Greek culture.

### 24. C
This question tests the reader's summarization skills. The test for question choice C is pulled straight from the paragraph, but is not word-for-word, so it may seem too obvious to be the right answer. The passage does talk about Nike being the goddess of war, as choice A states, but the third paragraph only touches on it and it is an inference that soldiers destroyed the statue, when this question is asking specifically for what the third paragraph actually stated. Choice B is also straight from the text, with a minor but key change: the inclusion of the words "all" and "never" are too limiting and the passage does not suggest that these limits exist. If a reader selects choice D, they are also making an inference that is misguided for this type of question. The paragraph does state that the arms and head are "lost" but does not suggest who lost them.

## 25. A
This question tests the reader's ability to recognize function in writing. Choice B can be eliminated based on the purpose of the passage, which is expository and not persuasive. The author may or may not feel this way, but the passage does not show evidence of being argumentative for that purpose. Choices C and D are both details found in the text, but neither of them encompasses the entire message of the passage, which has an overall message of learning about culture from art and making guesses about how the two are related, as suggested by choice A.

## 26. D
This question tests the reader's ability to understand function within writing. Most of the possible selections are very general statements which may or may not be true. It probably is a student who is taking the test on which this question is featured (A), but the author makes no address to the test taker and is not talking to the audience in terms of the test. Likewise, it may also be true students read more than adults (C), mandated by schools and grades, but the focus on the verb "read" in the first sentence is too narrow and misses the larger purpose of the passage; the same could be said for selection B. While all the statements could be true, choice D is the most germane, and infers the purpose of the passage without making assumptions that could be incorrect.

## 27. B
The time limit for radar detectors is 14 days. Since you made the purchase 15 days ago, you do not qualify for the guarantee.

## 28. B
Since you made the purchase 10 days ago, you are covered by the guarantee. Since it is an advertised price at a different store, ABC Electric will "beat" the price by 10% of the difference, which is,

500 − 400 = 100 − difference in price

100 X 10% = $10 − 10% of the difference

The advertised lower price is $400. ABC will beat this price by 10% so they will refund $100 + 10 = $110.

## 29. C
The purpose of this passage is to persuade.

## 30. B
The correct answer can be found in the fourth sentence of the first paragraph.

Choice A is incorrect because repenting begins the day AFTER Mardi Gras. Choice C is incorrect because you can celebrate Mardi Gras without being a member of a Krewe.

Choice D is incorrect because exploration does not play any role in a modern Mardi Gras celebration.

## 31. A
The second sentence is the last paragraph states that Krewes are led by the Kings and Queens. Therefore, you must have to be part of a Krewe to be its King or its Queen.

Choice B is incorrect because it never states in the passage that only people from France can be Kings and Queen of Mardi Gras

Choice C is incorrect because the passage says nothing about having to speak French.

Choice D is incorrect because the passage does state that the Kings and Queens throw doubloons, which is fake money.

## 32. C
The first sentences of BOTH the 2nd and 3rd paragraphs mention that French explorers started this tradition in New Orleans.
Choices A, B and D are incorrect because they are names of cities or countries listed in the 2nd paragraph.

**33. B**
In the final paragraph, the word spectator is used to describe people who are watching the parade and catching cups, beads and doubloons.

Choices A and C are incorrect because we know the people who participate are part of Krewes. People who work the floats and parades are also part of Krewes

Choice D is incorrect because the passage makes no mention of people who do not celebrate Mardi Gras.

## Verbal Ability Part II – Vocabulary

**34. B**
**Heinous:** adj. shocking, terrible or wicked.

**35. A**
**Harbinger:** n. a person of thing that tells or announces the coming of someone or something

**36. B**
**Judicious:** Having, or characterized by, good judgment or sound thinking.

**37. B**
**Ethanol:** n. a colorless volatile flammable liquid C2H6O.

**38. A**
**Respiratory:** adj. Of, relating to, or affecting respiration or the organs of respiration.

**39. B**
**Inherent:** Naturally a part or consequence of something.

**40. A**
**Vapid:** adj. tasteless or bland.

**41. C**
**Waif:** n. homeless child or stray.

**42. D**
**Homologous:** adj. similar or identical.

**43. B**
**Obsolete:** adj. no longer in use; gone into disuse; disused or neglected.

**44. A**
**Rankle:** v. To cause irritation or deep bitterness.

**45. D**
**Reusable**

**46. C**
**Torpid:** adj. Lazy, lethargic or apathetic.

**47. A**
**Gregarious:** adj. Describing one who enjoys being in crowds and socializing.

**48. B**
**Mutation:** n. a change or alteration.

**49. C**
**Lithe:** adj. flexible or pliant.

**50. A**
**Resent:** v. to express displeasure or indignation.

**51. A**
**Immaterial:** adj. irrelevant not having substance or matter.

**52. A**
**Impeccable:** adj. perfect, no faults or errors.

**53. B**
**Pudgy:** adj. fat, plump or overweight.

**54. C**
**Alloy:** v. Mix or combine; often used of metals.

**55. B**
**Combustible:** adj. Able to catch fire and burn easily.

**56. C**
**Salient:** adj. Worthy of note; pertinent or relevant.

**57. B**
**Ulterior:** adj. beyond what is obvious or evident.

**58. D**
**Junta:** n. ruling council of a military government.

**59. C**
**Laggard:** n. someone who takes more time than necessary.

**60. B**
**Languid:** adj. lacking enthusiasm, strength or energy.

## Section II – Math

**1. D**
$x^2 + 4x = 5$, $x^2 + 4x - 5 = 0$, $x^2 + 5x - x - 5 = 0$, factoring $x(x + 5) - 1(x + 5) = 0$, $(x + 5)(x-1)=0$. $x + 5 = 0$ or $x - 1 = 0$, $x = 0 - 5$ or $x = 0 + 1$, $x = -5$ or $x = 1$, either b or c.

**2. C**
Open parenthesis: $2a + 2b = 4ab$, divide both sides by $2 = a + b = 2ab$ or $a + b = ab + ab$, therefore $a = ab$ and $b = ab$, therefore $a = b$.

**3. B**
Let the XY represent the initial number, $X + Y = 12$, $YX = XY+ 36$, Only b = 48 satisfies both equations above from the given choices.

**4. B**
Number of absent students = 83 – 72 = 11

Percentage of absent students is found by proportioning the number of absent students to the total number of students in the class = (11 * 100)/83 = 13.25

Checking the answers, we round 13.25 to the nearest whole number: 13%

**5. B**
Let the father's age=Y, and Kate's age=X, therefore Y=32+X, in 5yrs y=5x, substituting for Y will be 5x = 32+X, 5x – x = 32, 4X=32, X= 32/8, x = 8, Kate will be 8 in 5 yrs time, so Kate's present age = 8 - 5 = 3.

**6. A**
This is a simple direct proportion problem:

If Lynn can type 1 page in p minutes,

she can type x pages in 5 minutes

Cross multiply: x * p = 5 * 1

Then, x = 5/p

**7. A**

First add all the numbers 2.5 + 9.5 + 4.5 + 1.25 + 7.05 + 20.8 = 45.6. Then divide by 6 (the number of data provided) = 45.6/6 = 7.6

**8. A**

This is an inverse ratio problem.

$1/x = 1/a + 1/b$ where a is the time Sally can paint a house, b is the time John can paint a house, x is the time Sally and John can together paint a house.

So,

$1/x = 1/4 + 1/6$ ... We use the least common multiple in the denominator that is 24:

$1/x = 6/24 + 4/24$

$1/x = 10/24$

$x = 24/10$

$x = 2.4$ hours.

In other words; 2 hours + 0.4 hours = 2 hours + 0.4 * 60 minutes

= 2 hours 24 minutes

**9. B**

First convert 350g to kg = 350/1000 = 0.35kg. Momentum of bullet = 0.35 x 250 = 87.5 kg x m/s towards target

**10. A**

To solve the equation, we need the equation in the form $ax^2 + bx + c = 0$.

$x^2 - 9x + 14 = 0$ is already in this form.

The quadratic formula to find the roots of a quadratic equation is:

$x_{1,2} = (-b \pm \sqrt{\Delta}) / 2a$ where $\Delta = b^2 - 4ac$ and is called the discriminant of the quadratic equation.

In our question, the equation is $x^2 - 9x + 14 = 0$. By remembering the form $ax^2 + bx + c = 0$:

a = 1, b = -9, c = 14

So, we can find the discriminant first, and then the roots of the equation:

$\Delta = b^2 - 4ac = (-9)^2 - 4 \cdot 1 \cdot 14 = 81 - 56 = 25$

$x_{1,2} = (-b \pm \sqrt{\Delta}) / 2a = (-(-9) \pm \sqrt{25}) / 2 = (9 \pm 5) / 2$

This means that the roots are,

$x_1 = (9 - 5) / 2 = 2$ and $x_2 = (9 + 5) / 2 = 7$

**11. D**

The cost of the dishwasher = $450

15% discount amount = (450 * 15)/100 = $67.5

The discounted price = 450 – 67.5 = $382.5

20% additional discount amount on lowest price = (382.5 * 20)/100 = $76.5

So, the final discounted price = 382.5 - 76.5 = $306.00

**12. D**

Original price = x,
80/100 = 12590/X,
80X = 1259000,
X = 15737.50.

**13. C**

Total hay = 214 kg,
The goat eats at a rate of 214/60 days = 3.6 kg per day.
The Cow eats at a rate of 214/15 = 14.3 kg per day,
Together they eat 3.6 + 14.3 = 17.9 per day.
At a rate of 17.9 kg per day, they will consume 214 kg in 214/17.9 = 11.96 or

12 days approximately.

**14. C**
125/100 = 1.25

**15. B**
The smallest prime number that can divide 125 is 5. 125/5 = 25. 25/5 =5. Prime factors of 125 = 5 x 5 x5

**16. D**
40/100 = 30/X = 40X = 30 * 100 = 3000/40 = 75

**17. A**
Momentum of first object = 2 x 3.5 = 7; momentum of second truck = 4.3 x 1.5 = 6.45. First truck has more momentum at 7 kg x m/s moving east

**18. B**
12.5/100 = 50/X = 12.5X = 50 * 100 = 5000/12.5 = 400

**19. C**
24/56 = 3/7 (divide numerator and denominator by 8)

**20. D**
The smallest prime number to divide 132 is 2. 132/2 = 66. 66/2 = 33. 33/3 = 11. 11 cannot be divided further by a prime number other than 11. The prime numbers of 132 = 2 x 2 x 3 x 11

**21. C**
Converting percent to decimal – divide percent by 100 and remove the % sign. 87% = 87/100 = .87

**22. A**
60 has the same relation to X as 75 to 100 – so
60/X = 75/100
6000 = 75X
X = 80

**23. B**
First arrange the numbers in a numerical sequence – 43, 45, 50, 65, 66, 69, 73, 75, 77, 80, 86, 90, 91. Next find the middle number. The median = 73

**24. C**
4.7 + .9 + .01 = 5.61

**25. A**
.87 - .48 = .39

**26. A**
Step 1: Set up the formula to calculate the dose to be given in mg as per weight of the child:-
Dose ordered X Weight in Kg = Dose to be given
Step 2: 100 mg X 23 kg = 2300 mg
(Convert 50 lb to Kg, 1 lb = 0.4536 kg, hence 50 lb = 50 X 0.4536 = 22.68 kg approx. 23 kg)
2300 mg/230 mg X 1 tablet/1 = 2300/230 = 10 tablets

**27. D**
Simply find the most recurring number. All the numbers in the series appeared only once. The answer is No Mode

**28. C**
4 x 4 x 4 = 64

**29. D**
5 ml/15 ml kX 1 tsp/1 = 5/15 = 0.3 tsp

**30. B**
To solve the equation, first we need to arrange it to appear in the form $ax^2 + bx + c = 0$ by removing the denominator:

x - 31/x = 0 ... First, we enlarge the equation by x:

x•x - 31•x/x = 0

$x^2 - 31 = 0$

The quadratic formula to find the roots of a quadratic equation is:

$x_{1,2} = (-b ± \sqrt{\Delta}) / 2a$ where $\Delta = b^2 - 4ac$ and is called the discriminant of the quadratic equation.

In our question, the equation is $x^2 - 31 = 0$. By remembering the form $ax^2 + bx + c = 0$:

$a = 1, b = 0, c = -31$

So, we can find the discriminant first, and then the roots of the equation:

$\Delta = b^2 - 4ac = 0^2 - 4 \cdot 1 \cdot (-31) = 124$

$x_{1,2} = (-b \pm \sqrt{\Delta}) / 2a = (\pm\sqrt{124}) / 2 = (\pm\sqrt{4 \cdot 31}) / 2 = (\pm 2\sqrt{31}) / 2$ … Simplifying by 2:

$x_{1,2} = \pm\sqrt{31}$ … This means that the roots are $\sqrt{31}$ and $-\sqrt{31}$.

**31. A**
At 100% efficiency 1 machine produces 1450/10 = 145 m of cloth.

At 95% efficiency, 4 machines produce (4 * 145 * 95)/100 = 551 m of cloth.

At 90% efficiency, 6 machines produce (6 * 145 * 90)/100 = 783 m of cloth.

Total cloth produced by all 10 machines = 551 + 783 = 1334 m

Since the information provided, and the question, are based on 8 hours, we did not need to use time to reach the answer.

**32. D**
Perimeter of triangle ABC is asked. Perimeter of a triangle = sum of the three sides.

Here, Perimeter of $\triangle ABC = |AC| + |CB| + |AB|$.

Since the triangle is located in the middle of two adjacent and identical rectangles, we find the side lengths using these rectangles:

$|AB| = 6 + 6 = 12$ cm

$|CB| = 8.5$ cm

$|AC| = |CB| = 8.5$ cm

Perimeter = $|AC| + |CB| + |AB|$ = 8.5 + 8.5 + 12 = 29 cm

**33. A**
10 x 10 x 100 x 100 = $1000^x$, =100 x 10,000 = $1000^x$, = 1,000,000 = $1000^x$ = x =2

**34. B**
$a + b + c + d = ?$
The sum of angles around a point is 360°
$a + b + c + d = 360°$

**35. C**
Simply find the most recurring number. The most occurring numbers in the series is 2 and 6

**36. A**
The scientific notation is in the positive so we shift the decimal 6 places to the right. Thus it is 5,630,000

**37. D**
There are 1000 mg in a gram. 30/1000 = 0.03 grams. To divide by 1000, move the decimal 3 places to the left. =

**38. A**
The shape is made of a square and a semi circle. Calculate the perimeter of each and add.
Perimeter = 3 sides of the square + ½ circumference of the circle.
= (3 x 5) + ½(5 π)
= 15 + 2.5 π
Perimeter = 17.5 π cm

**39. A**
There are 10 mm in a cm. 0.101/10 = .0101. To divide by 10, move the decimal 1 place to the left.

**40. A**
$2x^2 - 3x = 0$ … we see that both of the terms contain x; so we can take it out as a factor:

$x(2x - 3) = 0$ … two terms are multiplied and the result is zero. This means that either of the terms or both of the terms can be equal to zero:

$x = 0$ … this is one of the solutions

$2x - 3 = 0 \rightarrow 2x = 3 \rightarrow x = 3/2 \rightarrow x = 1.5$ ... this is the second solution.

So, the solutions are 0 and 1.5.

**41. B**
The formula of the volume of cylinder is the base area multiplied by the height. As the formula:

Volume of a cylinder = $\pi r^2 h$. Where $\pi$ is 3.142, r is radius of the cross sectional area, and h is the height.

We know that the diameter is 5 meters, so the radius is 5/2 = 2.5 meters.

The volume is: $V = 3.142 * 2.5^2 * 12 = 235.65 \, m^3$.

**42. A**
The decimal point moves 2 spaces to the left to be placed after 4, which is the first non-zero number. $4.5 \times 10^{-2}$ The exponent is negation since the decimal moved left.

**43. D**
The relation is the same figure rotated.

**44. D**
The shaded area is divided in half in the second figure.

**45. D**
The relation is the same figure rotated to the right.

**46. B**
The relation is the number of dots is one-half the number of sides.

**47. D**
First, we need to search for a constant common factor in each of the terms. If there is any, we need to take it out of the equation and write it as a coefficient in front:
$9x^2 - 6x + 12 = 3(3x^2 - 2x + 4)$

We cannot go further from this point, so this is the factored form of the polynomial

**48. C**
389 + 454 = 843

**49. C**
9,177 + 7,204 = 16,381

**50. D**
2,199 + 5,832 = 8,031

## Section III – Science

**1. A**
The formula for acceleration = $A = (V_f - V_0)/t$
so $A = (0 - 12)/60 \, sec = -0.2 \, m/sec^2$

**2. A**
The Law of Multiple Proportions states that when two elements combine to form more than one compound, the weights of one element that combine with a fixed weight of the other are in a ratio of small whole numbers.

**3. D**
All of the above are true. Electrons play an essential role in electricity, magnetism, and thermal conductivity.

**4. D**
An idea concerning a phenomena and possible explanations for that phenomena is an hypothesis.

**5. D**
All of the above. Chromosomes are

    a. Structures in a cell nucleus that carry genetic material.

    b. Consist of thousands of DNA strands.

    c. Total 46 in a normal human cell.

**6. D**
All of the statements about bases are true.

a. A compound that reacts with an acid to form a salt.

b. A molecule or ion that captures hydrogen ions.

c. A molecule or ion that donates an electron pair to form a chemical bond.

**7. D**
The circulatory system disease that is one of the most frequent causes of death in North America is heart disease.

**8. B**
Speed = (total distance traveled)/(total time taken)
X = 1000m/20 minutes
X = 50 meters

**9. A**
A chemical compound is a chemical substance comprising atoms from two or more elements in a specific ration as expressed in the chemical formula i.e., H2O

**10. C**
The plasma, or cell membrane protects the cell from outside forces. It consists of the lipid bilayer with embedded proteins

**11. C**
Protein biosynthesis is defines as, ribosomes synthesizing proteins in the endoplasmic reticulum. This process, also known as protein biosynthesis, is a process within the cell by which the substrates convert to products of higher complexity.

**12. A**
Cell fractionation. Fractionation is important because it purifies the cell and its parts.

**13. A**
The Strong Nuclear Force is an attractive force that binds protons and neutrons and maintains the structure of the nucleus, and the Weak Nuclear Force is responsible for the radioactive beta decay and other subatomic reactions.

**14. B**
Force = Mass times Acceleration Measured in Newtons.
1000 = 500 x A
A = 1000/500 = 2 m/s$^2$

**15. D**
Qualitative research deals with the quality, type or components of a group, substance, or mixture.

**16. B**
When a measurement is recorded, it includes the significant figures, which are all the digits that are certain plus one uncertain digit.

**17. B**
The equation E = mc$^2$ is based on the Law of Conservation of Mass and Energy, and states that Energy equals Mass times the Velocity of light $^2$.

**18. A**
A pH indicator measures hydrogen ions in a solution and show pH on a color scale.

**19. B**
Acids turns blue litmus paper red, base turns red litmus paper blue.

**20. A**
Covalent bonds involve a complete sharing of electrons and occurs most commonly between atoms that have partially filled outer shells or energy levels.

**21. C**
A base is any substance that can accept a hydrogen ion and can react with fats to form soap.

**22. A**
Water boils at approximately 100 °C (212 °F) at standard atmospheric pressure.

**23. D**
The dominant gene controls the expression of a trait.

**24. D**
Wavefunction is a mathematical function that gives the amplitude of a wave as a function of position (and sometimes, as a function of time and/or electron spin).

**25. B**
The vacuum of space is an environment where bacteria do not commonly exit. The nature of outer space, including intense cold and lack of oxygen, makes it difficult for even most bacteria to grow.

**26. B**
Plants and animals are kingdoms. There are six recognized kingdoms: Animalia, Plantae, Protista, Fungi, Bacteria, and Archaea.

**27. C**
Force = Mass times Acceleration Measured in Newtons.
F = 2000 kg X 3 m/sec$^2$ = 6000 N

**28. C**
A catalyst is a chemical involved in, but not changed by, a chemical reaction by which chemical bonds are weakened and reactions accelerated.

**29. C**
Organisms grouped into the **Protista** Kingdom include all unicellular organisms lacking a definite cellular arrangement such as **bacteria** and **algae.**

**30. C**
All of these statements are true.

A metal is a substance that conducts heat and electricity.

A metal is shiny and reflects many colors of light, and can be hammered into sheets or drawn into wire.

About 80% of the known chemical elements are metals.

**31. C**
The reaction of elements with low electronegativity(almost empty outer shells) with elements with high electronegativity (mostly full outer shells) gives rise to Ionic bonds.

**32. D**
AIDS (or Acquired Immune Deficiency Syndrome) is carried by a virus, not bacteria.

**33. A**
A collection of similar or like living entities. Class has the same meaning in biology as rank. Common classes or ranks include species, order, and phylum.

**34. D**
All of these statements are true.

a. Prokaryotic cells include such organisms as E. coli and Streptococcus.

b. Prokaryotic cells lack internal membranes and organelles.

c. Prokaryotic cells break down food using cellular respiration and fermentation.

**35. B**
Force = Mass times Acceleration Measured in Newtons.
1000 = 500 x A
A = 1000/500 = 2 m/s$^2$

**36. B**
The process of converting observed phenomena into data is called measurement.

**37. A**
The Law of Multiple Proportions states that when two elements combine to form more than one compound, the weights of one element that combine with a fixed

weight of the other are in a ratio of small whole numbers.

**38. A**
Morphology is the field that studies the relationship between structures in living organisms.

**39. A**
The mass number of an atom is the total number of particles (protons and neutrons) that make it up.

**40. A**
All of the statements are true.

    a. Mechanical energy is the energy that is possessed by an object due to its motion or due to its position.

    b. Mechanical energy can be either kinetic energy (energy of motion) or potential energy (stored energy of position).

    c. Objects have mechanical energy if they are in motion

**41. D**
In Eukaryotic cells, the cell cycle is the cycle of events involving cell division, including mitosis, cytokinesis, and interphase.

**42. B**
The atomic number of an element equals the number of protons in an atomic nucleus, and, along with the element symbol is one of two alternate ways to label an element.

**43. A**
pH is a measure of effective concentration of hydrogen ions in a solution, and is approximately related to the molarity of H+ by pH = - log [H+]

**44. B**
Ribonucleic acid (RNA) is a chain of nucleotides that plays an important role in the creation of new proteins.

**45. C**
Force = Mass times Acceleration Measured in Newtons.
F = 200 X 5 = 1000 N

**46. D**
The Law of Definite Proportions states that every chemical compound contains fixed and constant proportions (by weight) of its constituent elements.

**47. B**
Four factors that affect rates of reaction are: Temperature, particle size, concentration, and the presence of a catalyst.

**48. C**
Spherical bacteria are Cocci. Along with bacilli, this is one of the two major structures for bacteria.

**49. A**
A practical test designed with the intention that its results will be relevant to a particular theory or set of theories is an experiment.

**50. B**
The formula for calculating molarity when the moles of the solute and liters of the solution are given is = moles of solute/ liters of solution.
Moles of Solute = 3 moles of sugar
Solution liters = 3 liters
Molarity of solution = ?

Therefore: molarity of the solution = 3 moles of solvent/ 2 liters of solution = 1.5 M solution.

**51. D**
All of the statements are true.

    a. Electrically charged matter is influenced by, and produces, electromagnetic fields.

    b. Electric current is a movement or flow of electrically charged particles.

    c. Electric potential is a fundamental interaction between the magnetic field and the presence and motion of an electric charge.

**52. C**
Covalent or ionic bonds are considered "strong bonds."

**53. C**
P = 1.5 x 18 = 27 kg x m/s into the field.

**54. A**
Momentum of first object = 2 x 3.5 = 7; momentum of second truck = 4.3 x 1.5 = 6.45. First truck has more momentum at 7 kg x m/s moving east.

**55. D**
Reliability refers to the measure of an experiment's ability to yield the same or compatible results in different clinical experiments or statistical trials.

**56. A**
Genes are made from a long molecule called DNA, which is copied and inherited across generations. DNA is made of simple units that line up in a particular order within this large molecule. The order of these units carries genetic information, similar to how the order of letters on a page carries information. The language used by DNA is called the genetic code, which lets organisms read the information in the genes. This information is instructions for constructing and operating a living organism.

**57. A**
A higher concentration of reactants causes more effective collisions per unit time, leading to an increased reaction rate.

**58. C**
Each chemical element has a unique atomic number representing the number of protons in its nucleus.

**59. D**
All of these statements are about nonmetals are true.

    a. A nonmetal is a substance that conducts heat and electricity poorly.

    b. Most known chemical elements are nonmetals.

    c. A nonmetal is brittle or waxy or gaseous.

**60. B**
Moles of solute = ? or X
Solutions liters = 5 liters
Molarity of solution = 0.5 M
Therefore:   X moles/5 liters of solution = 0.5 or X/5 = 0.5
So X = 5/0.5
X = 2.5
Mole of salt in the solution is 2.5 moles

**61. A**
A solution with a pH value of less than 7 is acid.  A pH value of 7 is neutral.

**62. D**
Wavelength is defined as the distance between adjacent peaks (or adjacent troughs) on a wave.

**Note:** Varying the wavelength of light changes its color; varying the wavelength of sound changes its pitch.

**63. D**
First convert 500 g to kg = 500/1000 = 0.5 kg, momentum = 0.5 x 3.5 = 1.75 kg x m/s along the road.

**64. B**
A catalyst is never changed in a chemical reaction.

**65. A**
The prediction that an observed difference is due to chance alone and not due to a systematic cause; this hypothesis is tested by statistical analysis, and accepted or rejected is the **null hypothesis**.

**66. C**

In science and engineering, the **accuracy** of a measurement system is the degree of closeness of measurements of a quantity to its actual (true) value.

**67. B**

The horizontal rows from right to left of the periodic table are known as periods and elements on a row share the same number of electron shells.

**68. D**

All of the statements about solubility are correct.

    a. The solubility of a substance is its concentration in a saturated solution.

    b. Substances with solubilities much less than 1 g/100 mL of solvent are usually considered insoluble.

    c. A saturated solution is one which does not dissolve any more solute.

**69. A**

A valence shell is the shell corresponding to the highest value of principal quantum number in the atom.

**70. C**

To calculate the Molarity of a solution when the solute is given in grams and the volume of the solution is given in milliliters, you must first **convert grams to moles, and convert volume of solution in milliliters to liters.**

**71. C**

Hydrogen is the first element listed on the periodic table. The atomic number for hydrogen is 1.

**72. B**

Vertical columns on the periodic table are called groups. There are 18 groups on the table. Elements in the same group have the same number of electrons on their outermost shell.

**73. B**

The **range** of a distribution is the difference between the maximum value and the minimum value.

**74. B**

Formula - P= kg x m/s
= 35kg x 220 m/s
= 7700 kg x m/s east

**75. C**

A and B are correct.
An acid is a compound containing detachable hydrogen ions.
An acid is a compound that can accept a pair of electrons from a base.

# Practice Tests 3 & 4

Join us online for over 340 more practice questions (completely FREE) including a timed PAX Test to get ready for the real thing!

Go to https://courses.test-preparation.ca/course?courseid=pax3-4 and use coupon PAX34

# Conclusion

CONGRATULATIONS! You have made it this far because you have applied yourself diligently to practicing for the exam and no doubt improved your potential score considerably! Getting into a good school is a huge step in a journey that might be challenging at times but will be many times more rewarding and fulfilling. That is why being prepared is so important.

Study then Practice and then Succeed!

**Good Luck!**

## Register for Free Updates and More Practice Test Questions

Register your purchase at https://www.test-preparation.ca/register/ for fast and convenient access to updates, free test tips and more practice test questions.

# Online Resources

**How to Prepare for a Test - The Ultimate Guide**

https://www.test-preparation.ca/prepare-test/

**Learning Styles - The Complete Guide**

https://www.test-preparation.ca/learning-style/

**Test Anxiety Secrets!**

https://www.test-preparation.ca/test-anxiety/

**Time Management on a Test**

https://www.test-preparation.ca/time-management/

**Flash Cards - The Complete Guide**

https://www.test-preparation.ca/flash-cards/

**Test Preparation Video Series**

https://www.test-preparation.ca/test-video/

**How to Memorize - The Complete Guide**

https://www.test-preparation.ca/memorize/

**Online Library of Student Tips and Strategies**

https://www.test-preparation.ca/students-say/

www.ingramcontent.com/pod-product-compliance
Lightning Source LLC
Chambersburg PA
CBHW081354070526
44583CB00020B/2549